COMING TO TERMS WITH REALITY

HIDING BEHIND EATING DISORDERS AND
BORDERLINE PERSONALITY DISORDER

HOLLY CHINNERY

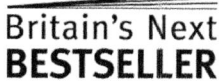

Britain's Next
BESTSELLER

First published in 2021 by:

Britain's Next Bestseller

An imprint of

Live It Ventures LTD

126 Kirkleatham Lane, Redcar.

Cleveland.

TS10 5DD

www.bnbsbooks.co.uk

@BNBSbooks

Cover design: Miacello©

ISBN - 978-1-914907-13-5

Printed in the U.K

With thanks to my friends and family, who without their support I may not have had the opportunity to see the other side and write about my journey.

Special dedications go to my husband Samuel, twin brother Steven and best friend Gemma for their extra special continued support, then and now.

What can you do when you are five years old and have the realisation that you will either become a serial killer or a nun?

This is my story of a life filled with mental health illness. As such it may not be a true reflection of other peoples' character and actions.

PROLOGUE

IT'S BEEN FOURTEEN YEARS.

Ten of which have been filled with numerous psychological treatments Now it's time. Time to finally say goodbye to you. Am I ready?

Not to rush a process that would inevitably lead to another relapse, I begin the farewell journey by writing a 'Am I ready to let go' letter.

 Dear ED,

This is meant to be a goodbye letter, but how am I supposed to say goodbye to you without saying goodbye to my existence? As a pre-teen the numerous failing attempts at changing my personality to fit in with people and situations saw you enter and become stronger in my orbit. My fragile sense of self-worth was escalating with the trails of navigating my teenage years. Weekends of food-restriction, secretive diet pill and exercise regimes as well as increasing episodes of binge-eating blighted me for the next four years. My one remaining ray of light in the form of University proved to be false hope. Having a more profound negative impact on everyone I met, you convinced me that the only way I could remain alive was if you took the reins. After all, what is the point of living when all I do is cause distress, or even worse, make absolutely no (positive) difference to anything?

The short period of rest I thought you were offering me has so far turned into 14 years.

Having to fight you is excruciatingly exhausting, especially when you've kept all of your promises.

Within two months of your full take over, I saw an enchanting personality that attracted others to me come out. The attempt to replace you with myself only lasted a few months when (perceived negative) changes to my social world and weight increase saw me run back into your arms.

Your impatience and need to take control ended a three-year cycle of you and I taking the lead of my body and mind.

Anorexia hit hard, but oh, what joy and elation it bought, especially when my life had to be put on hold.

Your physical manifestation bought with it love, care, support and attention from others: everything that I had been crying out for. Yet guilt engulfed me. With a preference to cause myself harm rather than others, I decided to recover and find another way to live.

Not so easy, you whispered to me.

The doubling of weight that occurred within the first term of returning to University saw you change tactics. For now, goodbye Anorexia, hello Bulimia.

Unable to expel enough from my body for your satisfaction coupled with a perception of recovery from others due to my normal weight, the toxic world of self-harming and suicide attempts came whirling in. But that was okay, as I still had you by my side and as long as I continued to have a bad, (bordering on the lines of dangerous), relationship with food, then my existence will be safe.

So the following four years was a mind-spin of intermittent food restriction, bingeing, self-induced vomiting, cutting and overdosing.

The 'If this is what I have to do to survive, then so be it' mantra that you fed to me day in, day out became tiresome.

Somehow achieving a long-held dream of mine led me to question my need of you.

After three months of going back and forth with you, I took the plunge.

The healthy eating and exercise program resulted in weight loss that was well maintained for two years.

Not to be.

The low humming that you provided for those two years was actually you taking time to further nourish the already embedded seeds you had planted. Taking advantage of a situation that ignited one of my greatest vulnerabilities, you swept me up and pulled me into your grips more tightly than before.

The daily exercises became obsessive and out of control. Allowing only certain foods into my body and only at certain times, the rules soon became coupled with the energetic return of self-induced vomiting.

Taking your revenge a step further, you toyed with my physical health for the first time.

With some fight left in me and from years of treatment, my eyes started to open to you being a false promise. I started to see the truth. That you have never been and never will be able to keep me alive. The only way you hold my existence in your hands is by having the power to take it away, not to keep it.

I am currently on top of the over-exercising, have stopped making myself sick, and become more flexible in the types of food I will eat. Yet your grip is still strong with restrictive eating now taking hold.

Standing in front of two doors, I have a decision to make. You, who can offer me immediate comfort but a bleak future. Or me, where an unknown path awaits but one that screams life.

With you so closely tied to my existence, turning my back on you fills me with fear and dread.

Am I ready to say goodbye to you?

I want to. Desperately want to. But I am not sure.

Yours faithfully,

Holly

PATHWAY TO DIAGNOSIS:

What can you do when you feel you were born into a world you don't fit into?

A world where you always seem to be two steps behind.

Where you feel you are floating high above everything and everyone – in a place of peace and tranquillity.

Yet, you want your feet firmly on the ground, feeling everything there is to feel and not being scared to.

Have the confidence, strength, certainty and faith to experience the power of emotions.

EMOTIONS – THE TRUEST ESSENCE OF HUMAN NATURE
THE VERY THING THAT YOU LOVE.

The thing that has the power to connect you with others.

I want it.

I can have it.

But I won't let myself experience it.

WHY?

Ever since I was a young girl I knew that there was something not quite right with me.

Being one of eight children you would think that I would feel some sort of similarity to my siblings; whether we were close or not. Yet, all I felt was a horrible feeling of disconnect, even estrangement. Whilst the others appeared to adapt to any given situation, I felt increasingly out of place. Even my sister with Asperger's appeared unfazed by life. These feelings were made harder to deal with by having a twin whereby people felt a free entitlement to compare us to one another.

Whether the comparison was as evident as I thought or was accentuated by my imagination, the despair it ignited in me remained real.

━━━

I have a childhood full of memories.

Memories of times where I have felt connected and of times where I felt disconnected.

First day of pre-school I was distraught at Mum's plan to

leave us there. Refusing to be separated from her, staff tried to entice me with different play areas. When it became apparent that this wasn't working, I was taken over to paint with my twin, Steven who was 'having fun.' Turning around to silently plea with Mum, I saw her sneaking out the back door.

Not knowing if she was going to come back I was consumed with feelings of inadequacy, rejection and abandonment.

Taking us two sets of the twins to the park, I overheard Nan telling Mum what sort of foods she should be feeding us.

What was going on here?

Was Nan telling Mum what to do? Did she think Mum wasn't doing a good enough job?

How dare she think that about my Mum!

Or, is there an underlying motive here? Did Nan say it within my hearing range on purpose?

She must have. But why?

There could only be one reason ...

She thought I was fat.

No, worse than that... she knew I was fat.

Even worse than that, I was repulsive and she had no strong feelings, or any feelings at all towards me. I was unworthy. Unworthy of love and kindness. And it needed to be known. Not only to me, but to everyone around me.

I needed to know the truth...

A day trip to Hastings, I took the plunge and asked Mum if I was fat. Her response that I would grow out of my puppy fat did nothing to deter the disgust I felt about myself.

Still in single digits the seed was sown. Set in stone. I was fat, worthless, disgusting, a failure. The list goes on.

It wasn't like I could convince myself that it was just my family who saw me that way.

As a twin, being compared to Steven was all I knew. It

didn't really ignite much feeling in me. That was until at Sunday School, where we were asked who was the bad twin and who was the good twin.

They must have known

But how?

Did my family tell them?

Or was it that obvious?

It must be obvious.

Were they being sly in telling me that I was the bad twin?

I just didn't understand … I just couldn't understand … What had I done?

I knew I was lost. I felt alone. I was scared. I was unsure. I was frightened.

I needed stability. The type that comes from feeling connected with others. But all the evidence pointed to me being discontented from others.

Why?

I must be doing something wrong.

Am I not expressing myself?

Do I need to let people know how I'm feeling?

How?

And can I risk that?

Not only would I be putting myself on the line without knowing the outcome, I could make my very fragile reality worse.

Engulfed by the pressure to label myself both externally and internally negatively led me to act that way.

As twins (Julie, Laura, Steven and I), we loved playing together. I suggested a game of seeing who would be able to walk down the stairs with their limbs tied up. Thinking it was doable, the surprise at seeing Laura falling headfirst down the stairs into the shoe rack with her glasses flying off, saw me immediately place the blame onto the other two.

Despite all three blaming me, no punishment was handed out. Nor was any further discussion of it.

Upping my game:

> *I refused to talk to Nan whenever she was over.*
> *I would threaten Mum with calling Childline for*
> *   cooking food I didn't want.*
> *I defaced household items often swearing at Mum.*
> *I would constantly blame my siblings for things I had*
> *   done.*

What did all this achieve?

Being labelled as a child with an attitude problem.

A child that can't be trusted, or believed.

A child that therefore feels disconnected.

Yet, this is not all of my childhood experiences.

There were times where I felt part of something ... where I was wanted ... where I was helped ... where I was encouraged. Times which filled me with warmth and fuzziness.

These times simply added to my confusion.

Summer days spent outside playing with my siblings and the other children on the street.

Family holidays to Great Yarmouth.

Playing cats-cradle with Mum.

Being a sixer at Brownies and being honoured by the vicar at Church.

Going to work with Dad on the trains.

Having a tight-knit group of friends during my school years.

Mum and Dad helping me afford my month trip abroad during school holidays.

⸺

These experiences led me to question myself.

> *Who am I?*
> *What am I?*
> *Am I a good person?*
> *Am I a bad person?*
> *Am I whoever people want me to be?*
> *Wait…*
> *Am I defined by people?*

That must be it.

I am the same person, yet I am received differently by people, dependent on how they are.

Therefore, to feel connected I must be what they need me to be.

I must fit into their ideal.

I must be good.

I must be perfect.

Their version of perfect.

DYING TO BE FREE

Insight afforded by the transition from child to teenager, saw benevolence replacing spitefulness.

A hectic household where compliance is heavily weighted filled me with a guilt complex. Labelling myself as the negative entity began the fight for perfection. By observing my parent's relationship, I became acutely aware of my effect on it. A word spoken at the wrong time, my presence unwanted, questions needing answering, all became added stressors to their relationship. Self re-intervention where positive acclamation is denied and negative identification intensified became the solution to life's woes.

Battling the burning desire to act out from the unconscious need for love required an exhausting amount of effort. Finally, instinct gave way to my head and heart with priority of self being transferred to others. My individuality faded away with feelings of unjust alteration.

Existing to everyone's own manual left me with a distorted sense of reality. In order to gain the recognition desperately desired, dissociative symptoms materialised from emotional detachment of social norms. Ignoring the urge to participate in primitive behaviours and consistently placing myself at the cost end of the cost and benefit scale saw failure to learn, accept and engage in appropriate self-desire. The resulting delay in gratification and social maturity not being learnt, led to the development of tunnel vision in my wants.

Foolishness in believing no harm would come of this enabled the 'Id complex' to remain the dominant psyche. Feeling like a non-entity desperate for some kind of acknowledgement, my fight to come out on top in all situations was filled with chronic second guessing. A proneness to gullibility resulted in excessive belief modification in light of novel information. Acting against all instincts propels me as the moments' desire by fine tuning the subtle variations in a given situation.

Firmly fixated in the narcissistic mind-set I delude myself that my uniqueness can only be understood by people with high-statues like my own. I become preoccupied with fantasies of unlimited success, power, brilliance, beauty and ideal love. Such a conviction magnified my feelings of right and wrong particularly when my want out shadowed the socially accepted norm. Enhancing my self-worth via the pleasure principle blinded me to the consequences that befell others, giving of the impression of an arrogant and haughty personality.

Amplifying the essence of human nature's heterogeneous relationship expands the manipulative hold over me. Acute sporadic episodes become daily occurrences due to the concentration of environmental cues and human emotions. The minds process of perceiving, discriminating, personalising and projecting information leads to registered stimuli producing deviations to prior responses. Failure in mentalisation payable to emotional naivety exaggerates these outcomes.

Heightened physiological responses generate an overactive imagination disabling the ability to search for alternatives. An automated visit to the pessimistic stance arises from the deficiency.

Depicted as being more crook, hindered my freedom from self-torment that others saw me as a failure. Internalisation of my pain soon became visible.

Give me peace in my heart, keep me loving,
Give me peace in my heart, I pray;
Give me peace in my heart, keep me loving,
Keep me loving till the break of day

A verse from a hymn that provided some comfort in times of distress

1

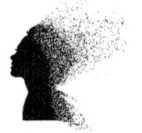

"Indignant at having to play second fiddle to the rest of the world, I took full advantage of separation from my family to regain some form of control.

No longer responsible for preventing dysfunction, I could now apply the control to me. Past expectations put to one side allowed for the much longed for inclusion.

Acceptance through desirability became a need worth fighting for.

The bittersweet taste of approval kept raising the bar. Genetically competitive, I would not give in until I succeeded. Flabbergasted at my ability to be so resilient made you a bigger force in my mind. Becoming a genius in perfecting myself to the utmost limit made me invincible.

I'M 18 YEARS OLD.

I'm moving 239 miles away from home.

From Kent to Plymouth.

Alone.

Albeit with Mum and Dads help.

I'm moving in with people I do not know. People who do not know me.

Starting a course with people I do not know. People who do not know me.

Attending many social events with people I do not know. People who do not know me.

I am about to embark on a journey of possibilities, choices and options.

Where everyone has a chance to start afresh.

To reinvent themselves.

To find themselves.

I am here.

At university.

As me.

Holly Chinnery.

Here is where Holly Chinnery will find herself.

Be comfortable with herself.

Accept herself.

Live for herself.

Welcome to the world.

I'm determined to find out who I am.

So I make a promise.

A promise to throw myself into every situation.

To say yes.

To see what the world has to offer and to see what my role in it is.

IT'S our first night in so my flat mates and I go for drinks.

Searching for common ground reveals that half of us are in relationships. Holding on tightly to this connection, I make my relationship out to mean more than it is.

To me at least.

After all we had only been going out for just over a month.

This little white lie might turn out to be true … given time.

More days and nights out with my flat mates follow.

Feigning a happy persona. A persona I want and think I can have, soon slaps me in the face.

Returning to our halls after a few drinks Becca and I join Jack in his room. Their flirting makes my presence unwanted.

No.

It makes me feel revolting.

It makes me feel like a leech.

I'm the third wheel.

The unattractive third wheel.

It's not like I want to be flirted with. I have a boyfriend. A boyfriend I'm loyal to. I just don't want to feel sidelined because I'm not good enough. Pretty enough. Because I'm unwanted.

I make my excuses and take refuge in my room. Where the darkness threatens to seep in.

Thrashing it away with a heartfelt pull of the cover over my head, I tell myself in no uncertain terms that tomorrow is a new day. I will start again. I will meet new people.

EXCITINGLY ANTICIPATING first day of the induction to my course I take time in preparing myself to ensure that I present the best version of myself.

Arriving in (assumed) plenty of time, results in me being

affronted with near on 200 people already seated, chatting away to one another like they have known each other for years.

Not only do I have to find an empty seat, which in itself is a challenge, the seat I find is next to a couple of girls who look down their noses at me.

Seriously, is there actually something wrong with me?

Frustrated behind belief, yet stubborn enough not to give up, I move after lunch finding myself with a group of people who speak to me. Ask about me. Make me feel welcome.

Finally.

The niggling voice soon sets in. 'You can do better.

You can find people similar in age to you.

People who have also moved away from home and living in halls.

People you can go out socially with.

People you can bring back to your flat and show your flat-mates that you have friends outside of them.

People who'll 'up' your own perceived standing.'

Feeling that I could better myself sees me become a person I don't like.

Having someone else join our group and being welcomed just as I was makes me feel hurt.

I'm not special.

She sits next to me in lectures and tries to make conversation.

I'm polite, but don't give much.

I feel conflicted.

I know I have warmth and compassion, but I'm not showing it.

I'm being rude.

I'm being a person I don't like and a person I know isn't me.

Then it hits me.

My course mates have treated us the same. Treated us with kindness, respect, interest and compassion.

They didn't judge me for the way I looked, for arriving a bit later, for the way I spoke, the fact that I wear glasses and have blonde hair.

They treat everyone like this.

The way that people should be treated.

As individuals.

And so I decide that the next day I will start again. I won't let my hurt be displayed in the way I engage with others.

I'll make conversation, show interest, even suggest going out for drinks as a group.

The very same day where I go all out to put my past wrongs right, I get dumped by text.

My penance is too late.

Numbness elopes me as does awareness that I need to react with upset, sadness and anger.

Being easier, I direct these feelings I was supposedly meant to be experiencing towards my now ex, rather than admitting that the fault lies with me.

Why does it lie with me?

Because, if I'm not who I am, then I wouldn't have been dumped.

I'm not worthy enough to be his girlfriend.

Probably not worthy enough to be anyone's girlfriend.

So, it's not too much of a leap to make the link that there must be something intrinsically wrong with me.

It's okay. I get it. It is what it is.

Unfamiliar with break-ups, I base my behaviour on what I think it should be.

A quick google search and recalling prior conversations

with friends and articles in magazines, I begin the 'too depressed to eat' phase.

First day of complete food withdrawal.

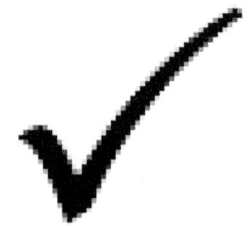

Not only do I smash it, it gives me more energy than a day of eating healthily and exercising.

With this much needed confidence boost, a new plan come to mind. One that I know I can do. One I will knock out of the park.

Wait for it...

Starving myself.

To achieve this, I need to keep myself busy.

So I spend nine to five weekdays on campus.

Evenings and weekends are spent going out, playing on the girl's cricket team, going to the gym and socialising.

Spare time is spent studying.

To avoid all temptation, meal times are spent far away from places related to food.

I DON'T PLAN on telling anyone.

This is going to be something I do on my own. An achievement that is all me. Something I can be proud off.

Yet, people knowing spurs me on more.

I can't let people down again. The suffering people tell me it will cause me is for the greater good.

Starving myself will free me.

It will turn me from a caterpillar to a butterfly.

The most beautiful butterfly that will ever be seen.

NEEDING something to live off and to fool that fat body of mine that it isn't being completely left out to dry, I decide to chew gum and drink coke only.

Thankfully. Very much thankfully, I'm still losing weight.

To top this success off, my feet are firmly in my course mates' social group.

Feeling invincible I push myself hard. Harder than I ever have before.

I attend all lectures, write up all my notes afterwards, undertake extra research, hit the gym at least 5 times a week, go out 3-4 times a week and do and be all I can for everyone I know and everyone I meet.

This includes taking steps to pull myself away from my ex.

So I burn the photos I have of him, delete his number, and stop listening to 'our song' on repeat for hours each day. Yet I'm not ready to let go.

Let go of starving myself rather than letting go of him.

So I message him online.

I'm certainly not expecting a reply, let-a-lone the one I get.

The metal plate in his head has shifted and he has a brain tumour. With only a few months to live I'm devastated.

I continue talking to him.

In no time at all the truth comes out.

He has slept with someone in fresher's week and he may not have a brain tumour.

His flat mates are blamed for spiking his drink the night he cheated, and the doctor's are blamed for him thinking he only has a short time to live.

I just don't have the words.

I'm drowning.

I knew he had many surgeries as a baby.

He told me to my face he had a metal plate in his head.

He had never lied to me. Why would he?

No-one I tell believes him.

That doesn't matter.

It doesn't matter that my school friend who is at the same University as him has seen him 'having a great time' on nights out.

It doesn't matter that I have a millisecond of doubt.

If someone confides in you, you believe them. You trust them. More than that you support them. You do all you can to be there for them.

To do that I need to be at my best.

To be at my best, I need to be the exact thing that he needs me to be.

———

ALL AT ONCE I'M thrown back to my early teenage years.

The years where I realised that by controlling what was going in my body I could modify my behaviour leading to a wanted existence.

Second term into year seven, a health professional turned up to school to take our basic measurements. Height of five foot one and weight of seven and a half stone saw me classed as being at the higher end of the normal weight range. Discussion of our results among my peers highlighted our differences. I was teetering on the edge. Both in terms of weight and socially. Maybe if I was that bit lighter, I would be that bit more socially included.

To be that bit more socially included I halted the many sporting activities I was part of, inside and outside of school. This way I could spend more time with my friends. To make sure that they didn't forget me.

The absence of exercise during the time where puberty was feared combined with the inability to dispel a three times a day habit (eating), saw consideration of other viable alternatives to maintain (with the hope of improve) my acceptance from others.

Secretly buying diet pills and weight loss enhancing exercise equipment proved futile. Excessively wearing the abdominal belt toner and taking more than the recommended amount of diet pills couldn't stop me from eating. Not when eating is very much a social activity.

Feeling dejected and without it being a well thought out plan, I decided not to eat for one weekend. Falling over bonfire night which was spent at my older sister's home made it seem that bit easier. Having gone the majority of one day without food, I was lulled into a false sense of security where no harm would come from having a little something to eat. It's not like anyone had commented or even noticed that I hadn't eaten.

Oh how wrong could I have been.

Not only was it noticed that I ate, it came to my attention that Mum had spoken to my sister to keep an eye on me as I hadn't eaten that day.

What the actual?

She did care. Mum actually cared. Cared enough to voice what I assume was worry.

I did mean something.

I meant something to my Mum.

I meant something... when it came to food.

29

The not eating food, part of food.
Okay, so this is it. This is what I got to do to be.
Think. Think. What now? What are my next steps?

⊏━━⊐

BACK TO MY EX...

There was no way in hell that I could start eating now.

This is much bigger than me.

Bigger than my need to lose weight.

I need to up my game.

Alongside spending hours in the gym, I jog around my tiny room, do 500 sit ups and 100 push-ups and star jumps per day. Furthermore, I cut my four 500ml bottle of cokes a day by half.

A grumbling stomach in lectures, weariness and a lack of concentration, dizzy spells in the gym and left arm tingling with a tightened heart muscle won't stop me striving for perfection. At the same time, the need for acceptance and belief makes Becca's appeal for me to see the doctor, one to be taken up. While I'm reluctant in receiving the prescription for anti-depressants and mineral and vitamin milkshakes, I'm more than happy to oblige in taking antibiotics for bronchitis and booking an appointment with the University's counsellors.

Why?

Because someone believes me.

They listen to me and believe me.

It doesn't mean that I'm going to stop what I'm doing.

Even though contact with my ex has almost diminished, starving myself has worked.

I was there for him when he needed it.

I did right.

In fact, I did good.

Now I need to move on. I need to continue this path, or at least maintain it to help the next person.

Definitely need to maintain it for Dads and Laura's imminent visit.

I worry what they will think of me when they see me.

What if it's not enough? Not noticeable enough.

What if they don't care?

What if they comment? Or don't comment.

Dad gives me a hug.

We haven't hugged since I was a kid.

Laura does her 'big smile' at me.

I don't recall the last time she smiled at me like that.

They mention my weight loss. It's obvious to them but not alarming. To them I'm slim but not skinny.

I feel confused.

I'm glad they've noticed, but why aren't they seeing it as a big deal.

The big deal that it is to me.

A few days later I go to the University's Counsellor. Her exact words that 'I'll be dead by now if what I was saying was true' stuns me into silence.

I'm not lying.

Am I'm lying?

I can't be. If it was just me to have witnessed this, then I could easily convince myself that I was lying. But I'm not. My flat and course mates have witnessed it. My family have noticed it.

But she's a professional. She must know best. She must only speak the truth.

Have I deluded myself into thinking that I have lost more than I have? Do I have a sleep eating disorder? Or, is there something about my body that means it won't shut down no matter how much damage I do to it.

I can't make sense of this.

I can't make sense of anything.

Some people say I've lost a lot of weight.

Some people say I'm not skinny.

Some people believe me and say I need support.

Some people tell me to my face I'm lying.

What the hell is going on right now?

Amongst this confusion I can't deny that starving had made me lose weight. By losing weight I'm able to be the best version of myself for others. By being what others need of me I'm being accepted.

It's this acceptance that gives my life meaning and a purpose.

⸺

IN ONE INSTANCE it all comes crashing down.

My flat-mates tell me that they don't want to live with me the next year. It doesn't matter that one of their Mum's will be buying a home for four people and with Jack moving in with his course-mates, and assuming I will move in with my school friend who was also at the University, it made sense to do it that way.

I have failed.

Worse than that, it doesn't matter what I do as I'll never be wanted.

Suffocating from this evidential thought and the ever nearing Christmas break where I will be expected to eat at home sees my mind start to accept the inevitable.

Somewhat reluctantly I begin to reintroduce food into my life. Not wanting it to dictate my social encounters, I vow to continue putting all my effort into other people.

Christmas is a revelation. I eat normally. I hang out with my friends … a lot. I work at my old weekend job. Laura lends me her old laptop to take back to University. Guys pay me attention on nights out, with a few trying to kiss me. Most surprisingly is that bumping into my ex at a club where he instantly transforms from sober to drunk when he clocks me, ignites no feelings in me.

Who would off known that eating and being socially accepted is not mutually exclusive.

Certainly not me.

Following my gut, I return to University with a new vigour.

No longer wanting to play on the cricket team sees me quit.

Knowing that being physically active is important for my wellbeing, I continue to attend the gym regularly.

Needing to eat healthily but aware that food is emotive and money tight, results in the decision to eat only one meal a day.

The main reason for being at University results in continual graft inside and outside of lectures.

Realising that I can have friends I do not see often, or even live with, I let go of the rejection that consumed me pre-Christmas and enjoy spending time with my flat-mates.

In fact, I start to realise that I do not have to have separate groups of friends. So I introduce my future housemates to my current flat mates and start to bring a few course mates over to my flat and invite them out. From this I also start to learn that it is also okay not to invite, or have everyone together all the time, whether they are part of the same social group or not.

I can see different people at different times and still be loyal to everyone.

With this revelation, I start to befriend other students on my combined course, rather than just those on my major subject.

This social growth cements itself on my last day at University before breaking for the summer. Seeing my friends pack up their belongings and go home fills me with sadness. Particularly saying goodbye to Becca who I feel a strong bond with.

It's now time to put an end to everything that has come before.

Time to move on.

To move forward.

2

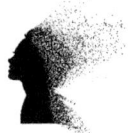

SECOND YEAR AT UNI – let's do this!

Put on weight? Yup. Who cares.

New Year, new start.

New housemates, fresh start.

Eating again. Yup.

Smaller room, paying less rent equals having money to buy food.

Healthy food.

Eating will prevent me falling into the same trap of marginalising myself from my housemates.

Eating healthily will hopefully allow me to lose a bit of weight giving me some social presence.

Wiping the slate clean with myself.

Wiping the slate clean with others.

⊏⊐

KNOWING I can no longer see things in black and white and that I need to stop taking an all or nothing approach, I begin to take a relaxed approach to life.

Well, to this year. See how it goes and I'll reassess.

With years of experience, quashing my initial reactions and emotions should take minimal effort. Of course, I will still feel, deeply. But as soon as an emotion hits I will label it and shove it into tightly bolted boxes in my head.

Starting with perceived negative situations.

It's the first day of being back and my school friend who I'm living with decides to return home and transfer University's so she can be with her boyfriend.

Not even twenty-four hours have gone by and I'm being abandoned.

Off that goes into a box.

It's the third day of being back and my old flat mates from last year invite me out for drinks that afternoon.

Am I betraying my new housemates by going?

Should I invite them as well?

Feeling guilty I also send this situation to a box in my head.

It's day five and my housemates and I meet the couple moving into the self-contained flat below us.

The guy speaks to us. Pays a lot of attention to Grace. Despite him moving in with his girlfriend.

God Holly, you are gross, they will never want to get to know you.

Off that goes to the deepest darkest box in my head. The one saved for times where I feel upmost repulsion.

Within no time at all, I'm able to throw absolutely anything and everything into a box in my head.

A month passes and a course mate tells me to 'pull my trousers up' as they keep falling down.

Well they better fall down, as I'm a size 16. 16 – Shocking.

Off that goes in a box of self-disgust.

Soon after that comment I am back into my small size 14 Miss Selfridge black trousers.

Oh, I do love these trousers.

That goes into my 'feel good about myself moment' box.

These boxes are allowing me to be unfazed.

Being unfazed means I do not over-emphasis things and am not consumed by things.

Things such as food.

Eating enough to function means that I am losing weight, but not dramatically enough to draw attention to myself, but enough to feel good.

Feeling good about my body allows me to perform socially.

And I am.

My course and flat mates' friendships from last year are continuing, I'm bonding with my new housemates and am making new friends on my combined course.

Controlling what I can whilst being indifferent is challenging, but it appears to be working.

Niggling voice: 'You think I'm going to let this continue?'

Uh-oh.

SHARING THE SAME BIRTHDAY, Grace and I decide to have a joint fancy dress party.

Desperate to enjoy the night and with the previous two months weight loss, I buy a size 12-14 'sexy' Dorothy Wizard of Oz costume online.

I should fit into it surely.

Nope. Still fat.

So, I stop eating, only allowing two Fiji milkshakes to pass my lips per day.

Two weeks later…still doesn't fit.

What now?

Returning home for reading week, Steven suggests I wear a white vest top over it. That way no one will see the zip at the back that won't do up.

With no other choice I go and buy a white vest top.

Utter shame and embarrassment.

Feeling consumed by inadequacies due to my hefty frame, I decide to get tipsy before people turn up at our house for pre-drinks.

I attempt to socialise but run out a few times, making excuses that I need to get something from my room.

That something being alcohol, which I drink quickly on my own.

Unable to self-soothe I look to others to take my pain away.

With everyone enjoying themselves, I focus my attention on strangers in the club.

It's not until the club is about to close that I find that person.

Josh.

Also celebrating his birthday, he comes up to introduce himself and wish me a happy birthday.

With not much time left, we flirt, kiss and swap numbers.

Ashamed at throwing myself at him, I decide not to text him.

A day passes. I feel weak, vulnerable and needy.

So I text. A 'it was nice to meet you' text.

Leave it at that Holly.

He replies.

Not to be rude, I respond.

We decide to meet up to get to know one another ... as friends.

Soon enough we start to date.

I try to ignore my gut.

Ignore the truth as not to feel guilty.

Guilty that I don't fancy him.

I fancy the idea of him. Fancy having a boyfriend. To show myself and others that I am wanted.

But I really don't fancy him. He's too nice.

Maybe I need a nice guy?

It would be a sign of moving on. From my ex, from feelings of inadequacy. It may finally bring me self-acceptance.

Doesn't that in itself make it worth a shot?

So I make a decision.

A head over heart decision.

To continue seeing him. To put my all in it. To fully invest in our relationship.

But it's not enough.

Not enough when it's just us, and certainly not enough when we are with other people.

I need more from Josh. Much more.

He may be sweet, kind, innocent and giving, but he is also geekish, childish and different.

Although I like that he is true to himself and unapologetic for it, he draws attention for all the reasons I don't want.

———

OVERWHELMED with guilt for feeling and thinking this way, I invite him to stay for a few nights at my parents' home over Christmas.

This will provide the opportunity for me to get to know him better, away from University.

If I'm being honest, part of me is also hoping that he won't like what he sees and decide to end the relationship.

Saving me the job.

So I unintentionally, but intentionally sort of plan situations that may make him uncomfortable.

Leaving him to speak to my friends and family on his own.

Seeing me get drunk and smoke weed with friends.

He raises no eyebrows and makes no comments.

He likes my friends and family. They like him too.

Right okay.

He is not what I thought he was.

Maybe my expectations of 'the Uni life' is tarnishing my relationship.

I'll start afresh with Josh next term.

Starting as I mean to go on, I take the lead in suggesting we sleep together for the first time.

I wonder if it will change anything.

It doesn't. Not for me. I still feel embarrassed by him, even the (I'm sorry to say, few) times when I look forward to seeing him.

For him, yes. He is acting more childish. Like he is in a toy shop or something.

I know that this should make me happy as it's an obvious sign that he is into me. But it doesn't. If you want the truth, it makes me feel a bit dirty. Dirty because I am using him.

I'M FED UP.

Fed up of being overly sensitive to people in my environment.

Fed up that this makes me socially inept.

So stuff it. I'll no longer recoil in horror when confronted with people and situations that I deem too good for me.

From now on I'll be an extrovert. A consistent extrovert that is not influenced or swayed by anything or anyone.

It starts and ends on Becca's playboy theme birthday party.

We play a game of 'I have never' before going out: the perfect opportunity to show my prowess.

I jump right in with an outlandish 'I have never' question knowing that someone will drink.

Next round, the tables turn on me.

I look at Josh to see his face covered in shock and upset.

It involves both of us but he doesn't drink.

Great, I've stuffed that up.

Later he tells me that he didn't want people to know.

Sleeping together a number of times in one night is not a big deal.

Fine, whatever.

I ignore him for the rest of the night, knowing that this will be the last night I can act extravagantly.

Trying so hard to fit in with others have once again proven to be my downfall.

A flood of memories come washing in.

Year 9 at school:

Somewhat idealising what I saw her life portrayed as, my attempt at mirroring Sharon produced opposite effects.

Eating two chocolate bars and a bowl of cereal after school, Sharon's weight remained stable whereas mine increased.

I completely ignored the fact that she danced 6 days a week and I had stopped all exercise.

While Sharon was the apple in her parent's eye, I was the maggot.

Didn't matter that this put restrictions on Sharon, and gave me freedom.

While Sharon's parents were united, mine with disjointed.

Knowing that appearances can be deceiving wasn't enough to make me feel better.

Year 10 at school:

Keeping a food diary as part of GCSE P.E gave me the excuse to go on a diet.

Feeling denied of the junk food my siblings were eating, I would sneak downstairs late at night or early in the morning to stuff my face. Whether I was hungry or not.

My need to fit in with others caused me to binge eat making me feel further ostracised from them.

I'M AT A COMPLETE LOSS.

A loss of how to be, who to be and when to be.

I find myself acting in opposites and at times, what feels like extremes.

Starting University, I refused to have an overdraft. Now I'm at its limit.

I used to start coursework as soon as it was given. Now I leave it to the very last minute.

I used to write up my lecture notes and revise as I went along. I no longer do either.

I used to be consumed with the need to have friends and lots of them. Now, I don't want them.

I would off given my right arm to be in a relationship. Now, I want out of one.

Outwardly I'm seen as functioning. Inwardly, I'm crumbling.

I no longer have one meal a day. I either starve for a day or binge on shop made food that doesn't require heating.

My decision to eat or not being based on my emotions. Unfiltered.

My decision to be with people or not, also being based on my emotions. Unfiltered.

The two together see's Josh's comment that I shouldn't eat junk food end our relationship. Me ending our relationship.

His sheer audacity is unbelievable.

The two together also impacts my ability to succeed.

Not able to stand being around people and needing to starve myself to fit (uncomfortably) into my sister's suit, sees me fail in getting the placement job. From the only interview I'm offered.

Oh well, I'm taking a year out anyway.

I'll sit my exams, go home and start again.

3

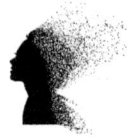

MINDLESSLY STARING at myself in the mirror I see a different girl to the one I know I can be.

Scared of my own shadow I'm constantly on guard, eyes flicking back and forth, pre situations played out in my mind.

Getting agitated, you pacify my 'withdrawing from others' guilt by providing dissociation tips. Memorising me with your charm, I let myself drift off into a dreamlike state where, I float between highly charged situations without being touched. In this tranquil place I am convinced that you have my best interests at heart. I feel protected and safe where I gain advice on dealing with life.

I've got a year.

A year to reinvent or find myself. For the third time.

Third time lucky right?

I apply for voluntary jobs. Secure two.

I continue to work part time in a supermarket.

I exert control over my food intake and exercise regime. Determined not to let the last two years of fluctuating weight and social standing repeat itself.

I set my alarm for half an hour before I need to leave the house as to avoid breakfast.

Quick shower, wash and change and I'm out the door. For the day. At least five days a week.

I either work or go the gym over lunch. Meaning there is no time for food. Only Fiji milkshakes.

I eat a salad for dinner. Unless I'm out with friends. In which case, no food.

It's working well. Really well.

Until my routine has to change.

I'm going on holiday to Malta. With my twin sisters and a mix of our friends.

I don't know what food will be available.

Plan A: I try to starve myself in preparation.

It doesn't work.

Plan B: I research where we are staying. Where food can be replaced with liquid.

I find a McDonalds close by.

Not ideal, but with little option, I tell myself that if I absolutely need it, then I can have one or two of their milkshakes instead of food.

They're similar to Fiji milkshakes right?

Unbeknown to me, we are met at the airport by a friend's parents.

Also unbeknown to me, they take us to their house for breakfast.

Crap. How do I get out of this one?

Me: 'I'm not hungry.'

Friends Dad: 'If you're one of those girls who don't eat then why are you still fat.'

I'm winded. Totally gob smacked.

Tears spring to my eyes and my body is poised to flee.

How dare he speak to me like that? Who does he think he is?

I'm going to prove him wrong.

So, I insist on spending a lot of time in his pub. To show him I have a fun personality, that is not related to food or body size.

I drink alcohol to help me achieve this.

I'm probably just making a fool of myself.

I also drink alcohol to blot out that I'm having a McDonald's milkshake **every** day, which I can't throw back up.

I'm a rubbish portrayal of an eating disorder. Can't starve myself enough or make myself sick.

I just want to go home.

I'm awash with relief as soon as the plane hits British soil.

I easily and happily fall back into my food, exercise, paid and voluntary work routine.

I go out more.

Visit Steven regularly in London, go to concerts, return to Church with Mum and meet up with school friends.

I remember that I'm allowed to have more than one friendship group at a time without appearing two-faced.

So, I also spend nights out with work mates and visit University friends.

What is this feeling?

Confidence?

Nowhere near.

Happiness?

No.

Feeling content?

Not quite.

Indifference?

Close enough.

———

I'M COMING up to twenty-one years of age.

Not having achieved the prestigious label of an eating disorder. After three years of disordered eating.

I might as well let it go now.

Now that I'm at a size that does not inflict any strong emotional response in me.

Right?

Steven surprises me with a haircut and colour and a make-up session at Selfridges in London for our twenty-first.

He then takes me for a photo-shoot.

Where he tells me to take of my glasses.

Where the photographers comment three times no less, that they will photo-shop the pictures.

This is not helping me.

I find myself having ideas of grandiose where Steven and I will be thrown into the limelight as the up and coming twin models. We will be idealized, seen as kind, caring, calm, perfect, serene and angelic.

I know these thoughts won't come true. I'm not that stupid. But they help.

They help pacify the anguish that our earlier birthday celebrations in Blackpool with his friends bought with it, as well as mentally preparing myself for going out in London later that night and my own celebrations back home the following week.

The copious drinking, clubbing, people's ability to adapt to situations (which I'm starting to learn is simply their enjoyment of this lifestyle), and the never-ending attention others are getting (primarily based on their looks) highlights differences. Differences particularly between Steven and myself.

Steven: skinny and attractive, is living in Central London, working at a well-paid job he got through a friend and is being treated to luxurious gifts and trips abroad.

Holly: fat and ugly, is living back at home having screwed up the first two years at University, struggling with life and self-punishing as a result.

With the gap between us too wide, I internally let go of Steven. I won't go anywhere. He knows where I am if he ever needs me.

―――

MOVING FORWARD INSTEAD of starting again

Well, isn't that a first!

I focus on getting the most from my voluntary work, pick up more hours at my paid job, increase my attendance at the gym, spend spare time with friends and plan and prepare for my two-month travelling trip.

Yet, I still feel an inconvenience to people.

It's Becca's 21st birthday celebrations.

We go shopping with her best mate the day before her party.

I really hate shopping.

They comment on my 'flat' bum.

My bum repulses me. It's a wrinkly satsuma.

Becca's Gran makes me a salad for dinner rather than insisting I eat the cooked meal.

I'm embarrassing Becca and causing extra work.

Three University friends cancel and the one guy already here is too ill to actually go out.

I've been deserted. How can I cope? Will I actually survive the night?

How bloody selfish of me.

Aware that Becca has been let down, I put every ounce of effort into hiding my feelings and ensuring she has a good night.

Not that it'll wash.

It doesn't.

I worry that I have sabotaged our friendship.

I worry daily for three months.

Until we secure a place to live for our final year at University. With three other friends.

⊏▭⊐

FEELING MORE secure in my relationships with others, I'm ready to go travelling.

I wave to Dad and Steven as I walk through airport security.

Vowing not to get caught up in my imperfections.

Telling myself that this is a fresh start.

That I won't make the same mistakes that I always do.

Mistakes with food and mistakes with people.

I meet a girl from the group the other side of security.

We have a few drinks.

She tells me what flight she is on.

I assume I'm on the same.

I look at my ticket. Realise that my flight is ten minutes before hers.

Oh shit. How can I tell her?

I don't. Not until the second to last call of my flight. Where I get my ticket out. Look at it. Feign complete surprise that actually, they are calling my flight.

I laugh it off. Make my excuses and leg it to the plane.

Idiot.

Still shaken, I pretend not to see the guy on my flight who I recognise as being part of our group.

Despite him smiling at me.

Nice one Holly. You could have used this as an opportunity to build a friendship before being thrown into a big group of strangers.

And to stop you getting lost at Bangkok airport for over an hour.

Undeterred, I go for dinner with two girls.

I order soup.

It gets picked up on.

One of the girl's comments that she knows people with an eating disorder, and it ruins everything.

How can me eating make her think I have an eating disorder?

How could she say that if I did, I would ruin everything? Was she warning me?

So, I begin to up my food intake.

To three small meals a day.

Determined not to let food dictate my travelling experience.

Niggling voice: *'Not that simple.'*

We learn to cook Thai food.

I can't do this. I can't be seen with food.

What if they make us try what we have cooked?

We arrive for lunch at a restaurant.

I see a handful of crisps on my plate, next to the sandwich.

I all but burst into tears and plan how I can catch the next flight home.

We stay at a Buddhist temple for a week.

No food is allowed after midday.

What am I going to do? How am I going to cope?

I skip dinner the night before a week long trek.

My body feels weird. My legs turn to jelly. I feel dizzy.

Oh my G*d, I'm going to die out here. In the wilderness. On my own.

We stay at a beach resort for a week. They give us food vouchers and tell us we can do what we want.

I eat three big meals a day and spend my own money on snacks.

Unhealthy snacks.

Lots of unhealthy snacks.

I've lost control. I've actually lost all control.

I'm disgusted with myself.

Utterly repulsed by my behaviour.

But there's hope.

I head to Ranong with five others to volunteer for a month.

Our three meals a day are cooked for us.

I can do this. I can reclaim control over my eating.

I can also start to form stronger bonds now there are fewer people.

Our first weekend off is spent in Phuket.

We go out both nights.

Everyone gets attention from numerous guys.

Except me.

I drink alcohol to loosen up.

It doesn't work.

I stand on my own. Pretend that I am fine. That everything is good.

But it's not. It's really not.

So I decide not to go away the next weekend.

Blaming lack of money.

Somewhat unintentionally, I stop eating.

I keep my body fueled with milkshakes and fizzy drinks from the small shop next door.

Until I am safely on the plane home.

⊏═══⊐

HAVING SURVIVED two months travelling abroad, not knowing anyone from the start, means the need has reduced greatly.

The need to pre-empt what people say and do.

The need to be ready for all eventualities.

The need to live according to my perceived thoughts of what people want.

Sometimes I am going to be a round peg in a square hole.

Absolutely nothing wrong with that.

I make a decision.

That when I am back at University for the final year, I'll say yes.

And I do.

I say yes to odd weekends surfing in Cornwall.

I say yes to joining the badminton club and debate team.

I say yes to spending days and nights out with others. People that I may not know well.

I say yes to things in and outside my comfort zone.

And I say yes to food. Particularly food.

I eat the two loaves of bread Mum baked for me.

Ignoring the voice that tells me to stop.

It's a voice of habit right?

I eat boxes of cereal.

Ignoring that voice once again.

I force myself to make a food shopping list.

A healthy but cheap shopping list.

With the plan of getting the food on it.

And cooking that food.

And eating that food.

CHAPTER 4

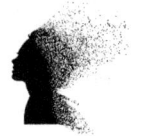

BAM

In a blink of an eye, four weeks have passed and all that has passed my lips are copious amounts of coke and chewing gum.

Nothing else changes.

I'm still being socially active and committed to my studies.

Though I see no issue or adverse effect in what I'm doing, my housemates do.

To be seen as doing, I go to the Dr's, make an appointment with the University Counsellors, get referred to the eating disorder service and have an assessment there a week before Christmas.

Yet again I feel unfazed. But this time it's without emotion.

Being emotionless sees time pass without incident.

Christmas comes and goes without eating.

Comments about me are made and not made. Neither evoke a response in me.

I know I'll get through this last year at University, but I don't know at what cost and am unable to visualise or imagine what will come after.

It's the third week of second term.

I'm struck down with gastroenteritis.

I drift in and out of sleep.

Am unable to hold down water.

Still refuse to eat.

My housemates tell me they are worried.

They take me to A&E.

I get an anti-sickness injection before being sent on my way.

They ask if they can call my parents.

My Dad turns up the next day.

Why is he here, trying to make me eat, insisting I go home with him and crying down the phone?

He has Asperger's. He doesn't show emotion.

I must be delirious.

I eat a couple of grapes and a lettuce leaf in front of him in an attempt for him to leave me alone.

He doesn't.

He's getting more emotional.

Oh for goodness sake!

Holly: 'Fine, I'll come back, but only until I'm over this bug.'

Up he gets, tells me to pack my bags and to be ready to leave at 8am the next morning.

Yes, sir! Right away sir!

I pull my covers off me, swing my legs from the bed to the floor and get up to pack my bag. *Oh shit. I actually can't stand up without falling back down.*

Crap.

How can I pack my bag let alone walk to the train station tomorrow?

All a sudden I'm crippled with fear.

━━━

Heading to the train station the next morning I cling on to Dad for dear life.

I make it.

I plonk myself on a seat with a sick bag in hand and fall asleep.

Getting off the final train, we get a taxi home.

Mum opens the front door and gives me a look of upmost disgust.

Dad drops the bags and calls the GP surgery, making me an appointment for tomorrow.

I don't need either of these things. I've obviously made a mistake coming back home.

━━━

I don't care that I have lost all but three stone and am underweight.

I don't care that I'm prescribed anti-depressants again or have to get a blood test and be referred to the mental health team.

I don't even care that the Dr advises Mum and Dad to cancel their holiday as I shouldn't be left alone.

I don't want Mum pacing outside the bathroom when I have a shower or the accompanying comments about how thin I am and that my stomach is now concave.

I don't want Steven coming down to have a go at me and talking to Mum about me behind my back. Especially because he is still skinner than me.

I don't want my parents telling everyone in the family about me.

I don't want to be at home.

At the same time, I don't want to go back to University.

I don't want to get help.

At the same time, every morning I wake up eagerly anticipating the arrival of an appointment letter from the mental health team.

I don't want anything, but I want everything.

The day the letter arrives, I rip the envelope open, see that I only have a week to wait, shove it under my parents noses and retreat to the front room to plan how to make myself more ill.

I don't know why.

It's the day of the appointment.

The phone rings. Mum passes it to me.

They cancel the appointment, rearranging it for two and a half weeks later.

I've got to wait another two and a half bloody weeks! Are they kidding me?

Two and a half weeks later I go to the appointment. It's at a different location and I'm being seen by a therapist rather than a psychiatrist.

That pisses me off.

She's nice. Tries to understand why I'm not eating. Pays me compliments. Gets me to think about my future, whether I want kids.

She suggests I go on a different type of anti-depressants and in the meantime she'll refer me to the eating disorder service.

Months pass with no news.

I'm still not eating.

I'm exercising every day.

My parents and the twins decide to host an intervention. They take my exercise equipment away from me.

As if that's going to make a difference.

There are stairs for cardio and tins of food and my hefty body for weights.

To shut them up I reluctantly agree to eat a slither of cucumber and have a smoothie a day with the aim of slowly increasing my intake.

Yea, right. Well, yea right to the cucumber and actual solid foods.

The fact that the smoothie is a liquid, sees my body and my mind force my hand.

I have a sip, which leads to two, three, four. Before I know it a whole glass of it is inside me.

I'm being disobeyed by my own mind and body.

Left with no choice, I put two fingers down my throat.

Can't even reach the back of my throat can I?

Slamming the toilet lid down, I sink to the floor.

I raise my knees to my chest, put my head in my lap and begin to weep.

Weeping, at once again failing.

CHAPTER 4

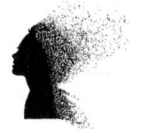

The deadly venom you excrete finds its way towards me assaulting my senses and attacking my emotions.

I beg at you to leave me alone. Your sight, your smell, your taste, your touch haunt me. You're in my dreams at night and fill my days with fear. You are the work of the devil who insists on tormenting me. I hate you but I crave you. I don't want you but I need you. You make me feel weak, vulnerable and alone whilst offering protection comfort and support.

I pace my bedroom floor, invasive thoughts of food running wild in my head. A constant battle with my conscious never returns a sound decision. Whilst my starving body cries out for food, my mind restrains me by use of scare tactics. The tremendous desire

for career and personal triumph makes
resistance futile. Success overriding
any of the momentary pleasure food may
bring ultimately leads to its exclusion.

For the first time there is nothing.

When I've been worried or anxious in the past, I looked to the future. I saw many possibilities and outcomes where I found peace with myself and others. Where I no longer based my existence on others.

Now? I can't even cope being in the moment.

As for my past, I can't make sense of it. It is eroded with darkened skies, treacherous storms and an abundance of terror.

Even sleep isn't enough to alleviate my despair.

Something does though... momentarily.

I jump out of bed in a rush for the toilet.

I sway, but continue making my way to the bathroom.

I hold onto my bedroom door frame.

I leave my bedroom and step into the hallway.

All a sudden I'm on the floor in the hallway with Mum standing over me.

I look up confused.

Dad comes rushing up.

I close my eyes again. Open them. They're still there.

Mums silent.

She's never silent.

I try to get up. Dad helps me.

I touch the back of my head.

There's blood on my hand.

Mum and Dad insist I go to the hospital.

I feel something. Not quite excitement or joy.

What is this feeling?

Hope.

The excitement and joy are the associated feelings of hope.

On the pretence of wanting to see the back of my head…

Holly to Mum: 'Can you take a photo.'

I pass Mum my phone.

Not as bad as what I thought.

I feel dejected.

I'm at the hospital with Dad.

The Dr asks what happened.

I say that I collapsed because I'm not eating and that I'm not going to.

She puts stitches in my head and tells me about her friend who is anorexic.

I get that you're trying to relate and offer me comfort but this is about me.

I need you to fast track me into the eating disorder service.

Stitches are done and she sends me for an ECG, blood and urine tests.

They all come back clear.

Damn it.

They discharge me.

Please call me back. Please tell me there was a mistake. Please tell me that I need to go straight to an inpatient ward.

I can't do this anymore. I really can't do this anymore.

Nothing.

I go home. It's half past one in the afternoon.

I've missed my first smoothie of the day.

I'm going to have to wait till four pm for the next one.

But I can't.

My routine has been screwed up and I don't know what to do about it.

Do I make up the lost one or wait for the next one?

If I wait, do I double up or just have the one?

Why didn't they just take me away?

━━━

Time continues to pass.

Emptiness continues to elope me.

My parents debate whether I should be allowed out on my own.

Mum to Dad: 'If she's going to collapse again then she will whether she's inside or outside.'

Ermm... ouch.

I don't want to be inside anyway.

Not when we have a massive kitchen with two fridges and freezers and numerous cupboards full of food. Where all I can do is watch TV that every half hour sees some reference to food being made.

Especially not when people come over, look and make comments about me behind my back or to my face.

Nothing is happening and my family are getting fed up.

That much is obvious.

Snide comments are made and easily absorbed that I'm solely doing this for attention, that University has caused my eating disorder, that I'm a drain on them all and they are better off without me. Well, that last bit I add on. But it's true.

Not wanting to owe them anything, I begin to sell my things on eBay so I can pay for my own smoothies and to self-fund a mini break away surfing with my University house-mates after their final exams.

As if that's going to happen given that I'm struggling to walk up the stairs without feeling faint.

———

I reluctantly go back to the Dr's for another prescription of anti-depressants.

The Dr weighs me and takes my height.

Dr: 'Have you heard from the eating disorder service?'

Holly: 'No,'

Dr looks at my notes.

Dr: 'You collapsed? Why hasn't anyone told me this?'

Dr finds a letter from the eating disorder service from a few months ago.

Dr: 'They rejected the referral as you did not meet the criteria.'

You mean they didn't think I was skinny enough.

The Dr seemed perplexed at this and at not being informed.

He sends an urgent referral back to the mental health team for reassessment. He states he will emphasis that I've lost another stone and a half, have collapsed and have electrolyte imbalance.

That strange feeling is back.

Hope.

I go home and tell Mum and Dad.

Hopefully they'll change their view that I'm a drain on them.

CHAPTER 5

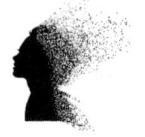

TICK TOK

TICK TOCK TICK TOCK

It's been four months since I've been at home and another four until the new academic year. I'm going back, no doubt about it. But I'm still not eating and I'm yet to hear from the eating disorder service.

I have no choice.

I have to start eating.

With the church bells chiming signifying midday, I make my way into the kitchen where Mum's cleaning the cupboards. My mental pacing turns into physical pacing. To calm myself, I sit down on my hands

It's now or never.

Holly: 'I might have a sandwich.'

Mum: Not looking up, 'If that's what you want to do.'

With deep breathes, I move the chair back and stand up. I head to the cupboard to get a plate. Then to the cutlery draw to get a knife. Next is the bread bin.

Don't think about it.

I remove two slices of seeded bread, placing them on the plate.

Okay, next.

Off to the fridge for spread and cucumber.

Mum: 'Do you want me to make it.'

Holly: 'No, I'm okay.'

Breathe. In and out. In and out.

I take the lid off the spread, pick up the knife.

You can make the sandwich, but you don't need to eat it.

But just in case you do, use absolute minimal spread.

I lay five slithers of cucumber carefully between the two slices of bread.

How shall I have the sandwich?

Cut in half?

In quarters?

As squares?

What about triangles?

How do adults have their sandwiches? In half. Straight down the middle.

Taking my plate, I sit back down, directly behind Mum.

I don't need to eat it all. I can have one half. I doubt my stomach will be able to handle much more.

First bite down.

That was easy. Much easier than I thought.

Oh wow. My plate is suddenly empty.

Holly: 'Finished.'

Mum: 'Well done.' Carried on cleaning.

I get up, wash away the evidence and retreat to the front room where I hide under the bedspread.

I actually ate.

Crap.

Why don't I feel bad about it? I need to beat myself up.

I've walked into my own trap. Mum now knows I can eat and will expect me to continue to do so. But that's okay.

No it's not.

What's for dinner?

What the hell?

An image of the bathroom scales pop into my head.

Extreme fear hit.

There's no way in hell I can weigh myself now.

Not hourly, not daily, not weekly, not ever.

But I need to know.

Know how much weight the sandwich has put on me.

No, I can't know. I don't want to know.

I'm upstairs, hand on the sink basin, staring at the scales.

It's the afternoon. I won't be at my lightest.

Come on Holly, you can do this. It will inform you whether you eat again or not.

I close my eyes, holding tightly onto the basin, put one foot on the scale.

I open one eye and look down. Okay, I haven't put on 12 stone in one half of my body.

I squeeze both eyes shut. I place my second foot on the scales. My knuckles turn white.

Breathe Holly Breathe.

Rip the band-aid off.

I fling my eyes open, look down.

Still under seven stone.

No increase.

I take a big sigh of relief.

Wait a minute.

I have just eaten. You don't put on weight immediately.

It could be hours, days, even weeks before I know the full amount of damage this mistake has caused me.

I'm left with no choice. I got to keep weighing myself.

Mentally preparing myself for the horror to see that scale go up a notch.

That blasted sandwich is doing me more harm than good.

I step of the scales, remove myself from the bathroom. I quietly go downstairs resuming my place on the sofa, hiding and thinking.

Thinking and thinking and thinking.

All that I can do as not to jeopardise myself any further is to see that sandwich as a one off and as a replacement.

Goodbye smoothies.

Three o'clock comes and goes. Slowly.

I look at the clock. Back to the TV. Back to the clock. TV. Clock. TV. Clock. TV.

I get up, put my ear to the clock.

Tick Tick Tick.

Check the time on my phone. It's the same.

Back to the sofa.

Flip through the channels. Nothing that grabs my interest.

Try to sleep. It eludes me.

Do some exercises. No energy

Read a book. Can't concentrate.

Walk to the kitchen. No one there.

Back to the front room.

Fuck this.

I'm in the kitchen, glass in one hand, smoothie in the other.

I pour. No more than a couple of sips worth.

Tip it down my neck.

Didn't want that.

Pour some more.

Tip that down my neck.

I do it once more.

I'm out of control.

Before I get caught, I put the smoothie in the fridge, wash up the glass and put it back in the cupboard.

What have I done to myself?

Two seconds later… *what's for dinner?*

Oh please God help me.

Before today I haven't eaten for six months – surviving on liquids.

I'd proven to myself that I don't need food. Now I've relapsed.

I hate what I've just done and I am beating myself up about it.

At the same time I don't wholly feel bad about it.

Confused about my feelings and unable to process them I go upstairs and climb into bed.

Oh no. No no no.

This can't be happening. But of course it is. And it's happening now.

The scales have moved. They have moved up in time for two events I'm going to.

So here is the deal. I am going to stop eating from today.

Three hours later… nope that's not going to happen.

Tomorrow I'll start again.

The next day.

Or the day after that.

Or even the day after that.

Is there an actual thing of new day new start or am I just fooling myself?

Not able to bear being in the same room as the scales and unable to remove them for fear of drawing attention to myself, I start to challenge myself in leaving the bathroom as quickly as I can. I time how long it takes me to clean my teeth, shower, go to the toilet and then try to reduce this next time. I will no longer weigh myself.

And I don't.

Not until a week before my cousins party.

Wholly petrified at what they will say to me but in desperate need to look amazing at this family event, I close my eyes and stand on the scales. Leaning heavily to the right with my hand gripping the sink, I slowly open one eye. Quickly shutting it before registration, I move my left leg to the end of the scales in a further attempt to alter my weight. Trying again, with my right eye open and my body shuffling to the edges of the scale, I read the dial with a tightening grip on the sink.

Shock and confusion that I have not put on any weight sees me shuffling nearer the centre of the scales and loosening my grip from the sink. Six attempts later, my whole body weight is on the scales with no extra support.

The scales indicate that my weight has gone up half a pound.

It's a lot, but it's nothing in comparison to what my mind has been conjuring up.

Someone must have adjusted the scales.

Carefully stepping off the scales, I readjust the dial making sure it is exactly on centre of the zero before nervously stepping back on. Again the same weight confronts me.

Maybe it's the location of the scales?

I move the scales around the bathroom numerous times.

I'm confronted with the same numbers.

Not wanting to be the fool in this mastery of someone's, I vow to continue with my substance intake but will weigh myself day and night, and if I notice any weight gain I will know that someone has been fiddling with the scales at this crucial time in my life.

For now, I will prepare for the party.

Prepare to be seen but not to be seen.

Prepare to be talked about but not talked about.

Prepare what I wear, how I'll enter the room, what I do in the night, how I interact with others, what my responses to questions will be.

Most importantly, prepare how I will cope in the change of routine and what this means for my inevitable food intake.

I want to make an entrance but I end up hiding behind my parents. I still notice the stares.

I want comments that are out of complete care and concern.

I get nothing. Not a word.

So I sit for a bit. I get up and dance (once) on another cousins insistence. I take pictures.

I guess I'm treated normally.

But I don't know what they think and I need too.

So later that night I go to bed knowing that I mean nothing to anyone no matter my size, shape or personality. My place on earth is a mistake and no matter what I do, I can't change it.

In a (failed) attempt to shake this thought, I blame my feelings of nothingness on my family.

Just in time to stay at a friends for the night and not have to worry what my family think.

Oh, crap. I'm going to be away overnight.

I can't let people see me eat.

I need a food plan!

Here it is:

First day away I will eat my sandwich before I leave - 7 hours early.

On the second day I will have the sandwich when I get home – only 1 hour later.

I know people will look at me so I have to be on form socially.

All I want to do is hide.

The social plan is to dress up in 80s gear, drink at their house then go out. So it takes me by surprise that they spontaneously decide to eat beforehand.

What students eat before going out to get drunk?

Oh crap. People I've never met before will know my secret.

They order Chinese.

They eat in front of me. Slowly.

Crap my stomach is rumbling.

Tick tock, tick tock. Time is all but coming to a halt.

I'm scared to move, scared to make a noise, scared to breathe.

I'm scared to go upstairs and change knowing that my outfit will no longer fit me, even though my top is a size twenty-two.

I'm scared to come back downstairs where people will see what I'm wearing.

Even though Steven pours my drinks so I have minimal alcohol, I'm scared to drink because of the calories.

I'm scared that I'm not good enough.

And I'm not.

Steven's mate who comes with us tells me that I should stick two fingers down my throat.

That's proof enough. Prove that I'm not good enough.

It is now summer and I still haven't heard from the eating disorder service.

Obviously I've been rejected again.

This combined with knowing I can't continue to sponge off Mum and Dad, not wanting people to keep moaning at me and having decided (because I don't have a choice) that I'll be going back to University, I resign myself to increasing my food intake. My one day cucumber sandwich will now include lettuce, tomato and tuna.

Then it comes.

Glistening on the door mat face up, wanting to be seen.

The letter I've been waiting months for is finally here.

I've been invited for an assessment at the eating disorder service.

Why wasn't I able to hold off eating for a few more months?

Straight away I decide to stop eating.

Yet again I fail.

I have a good few weeks to keep trying though.

And I try.

And I keep failing.

Everyday leading up to the appointment, I try my outfit on and weigh myself. With shoes on and without shoes on. With my coat on and without my coat on. In different locations and at different times within the two and a half hour appointment slot (which of course had to be in the afternoon when you are at your heaviest).

I practice standing in particular ways to ensure I'm at my lightest. I stretch hoping to grow that bit taller hoping that this will make my weight look less.

I spend hours planning and checking the best route to the appointment.

Of course we get stuck in traffic and of course I get weighed as soon as I arrive.

Two pounds heavier? You've got to be kidding me.

Holly: 'I weighed myself this morning, I was not that

heavy. The scales are wrong. It must be my clothes. Can we do it again.'

Staff member: 'Don't worry about it, the scales can be out slightly.'

Yea, right.

Having failed the physical test, everything is hanging on my verbal communication ability.

You will not reject me again.

Family background, personal history, how I view myself, and of course, food, are all discussed in great detail.

Three weeks later the assessment letter comes.

Last paragraph:

'Dr Bowles suggested that she thought inpatient treatment would be helpful for you but you felt that this was
not appropriate at the moment because you are very
keen to go back to University in September. You feel
strongly that you know your own mind and you know
what you want to do. After discussion at our team
meeting we feel that you could benefit from some individual therapy and you will hear from us again as soon
as a therapist is available.'

DID SHE FUCK!

I would have taken the inpatient offer up in a heartbeat. Absolutely, no two ways about that.

Wait a minute.

Oh G*∂, Oh G*∂, Oh G*∂, Oh G*∂.

I kept banging on about going back to University and saying that I was strong willed.

But that's not what I meant.

When I'm in uncomfortable situations I feel I need to prove myself. That was me proving myself.

Why couldn't they see that?

Second sentence of the letter:

'If there is anything in this letter you do not agree with please let me know and I will amend your medical records.'

Who am I to make a judgement on the letter. Especially from a health professional.

It's not right and its disrespectful.

So I don't. I leave it.

Maybe if I let Mum and Dad read the letter they may encourage me to call them back?

Not that I will let them read it. For fear of upsetting them.

It didn't matter now.

The decision is out of my hands. I'm to return to University in just over one month.

⸺

There's no point in anything anymore.

No point in not eating, no point in eating.

No point in living, no point in dying.

There is no point. No point in me.

I disconnect. Only engaging in basic human needs.

I shift my sandwich from night time to day time, allowing for the tiniest steamed white fish and vegetables in the evening.

I speak when I perceive it as necessary.

I go to bed and get up at decent 'normal' times.

I wash and change daily.

I maintain this up until a couple of days before I'm due to leave.

Mum: 'if you hadn't started eating dinner then I wouldn't have let you go back.'

What?

I only ate because I thought that was what you had wanted. For me to go.

If I had known that you would say this, or were thinking it, I would not have eaten, which by the way has made me feel incredibly shit and repulsive, and, I 100% would have called the eating disorder service asking to be an inpatient.

Holly: 'Okay.'

Maintained it for it to be thrown back in my face.

I give my everything. But everything is all for nothing.

CHAPTER 6

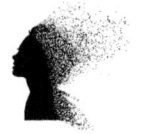

It's taken four years to get the diagnosis of Anorexia Nervosa.

A diagnosis that portrays my emotional distress.

And it's taken a mere few months to screw it up.

Well, thank you. Thank you very much.

Van's packed.

Dad's in the driver's seat. I'm in the passenger seat

Engine is turned on.

Say it, say it now.

Say you don't want to go back. Say you were offered inpatient treatment and that you will call up the eating disorder service and ask them to admit you. Surely they won't say no as it's been less than a month since you got that letter. Lie to them about having eaten more.

The van's moving.

It's leaving the street,

It's travelling through town.

On the A road.

Now the motorway.

No turning back now.

We are at a service station. Dad is in the toilet.

I quickly wolf down the sandwich that was meant for dinner.

For G*ds sake Holly, It's not even midday!

Dad's back.

We are not that far from home. Tell him you've changed your mind and you need to go back.

I can't. I don't know if the University will allow me another year off.

We are back on the motorway.

It's two pm. We've parked outside the house I'm living at for the next year.

A house full of strangers.

Definitely can't change my mind now.

I suck it up.

No one in.

Good.

Quickly dumping my stuff in my room, I force Dad and myself out the house so I can join the gym, make a Dr's appointment and to begrudgingly go food shopping.

I do plan to go to the gym. Hit it hard at least 5 days a week.

I also plan to go to the Dr's and get referred back to the eating disorder service to start the treatment I didn't get to last year.

But I don't plan to eat. At all.

Yet I eat.

I eat as soon as Dad leaves later that day.

I eat in spite of the signs telling me I don't need to.

The signs of forgetting the tin opener and having to rush out to buy one.

The signs that one housemate has already moved in and could return at any minute. And with that, the signs that three more housemates also unbeknown to me could come through the front door right this second.

Eating is a compulsion that brings absolute terror with it. A compulsion I cannot deviate from.

Yet I'm deviating from the other compulsion of not eating.

I feel panicked.

I can't sit with this feeling. I need to suppress it and fast. Food has always done that for me. But now as I have started eating I have no choice but to carry on. So I hurriedly make another sandwich, run upstairs with it and wolf it down.

That is now two massive sandwiches in one day. A monumental day, for I know it will go on to signify the day I let my mental health rapidly deteriorate.

⸻

Please help me.

Oh, please.

Someone.

Anyone.

Come take the control away from me.

Lock me up. Throw away the key.

Don't leave me here.

Come back.

Protect me.

Save me.

⸻

It's the first night in my new home.

I tell myself that tomorrow is a new day. I can and I will start again.

Gym

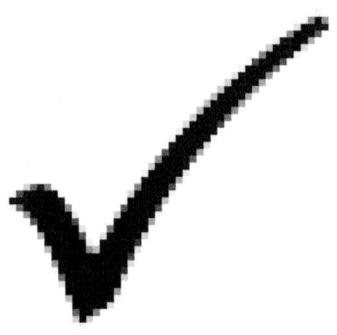

Dr's

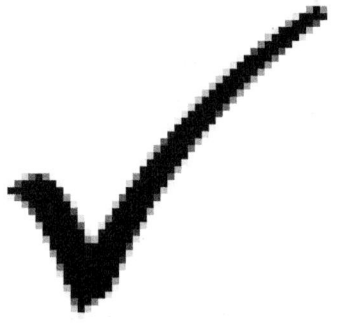

A referral back to the eating disorder service.

Food, should be a **X** but is a

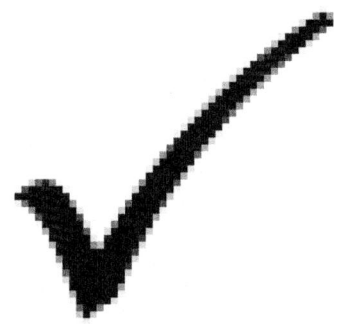

Well, that was a grave mistake.

Of course my house mate walks in when I'm in the middle of making my sandwich.

Of course he is with a group of friends.

Of course he comments on the size of my sandwich.

First impressions are everything,

Mine is now that of a pig. A fat, greedy pig.

Great.

I'm panic stricken again.

I want to scream and shout. Throw everything off the kitchen unit with one swipe of my arm. Run upstairs, throw myself on my bed with tears streaming down my face, howling like I've never howled before.

Instead I laugh it off, carry on making my sandwich, saunter of upstairs, eat the sandwich regret it with every bite and spend the rest of the time pretending that everything is okay.

This pattern continues.

On and on it goes.

Two gigantic sandwiches a day.

At least I'm able to go to the gym every morning for two hours.

Ha!

It starts with a day off from the gym.

I feel rejuvenated, refreshed and raring to go. So when my housemates asks if anyone wants to go to the shop with her to get milk, I jump up at the opportunity.

Not to buy anything myself mind you.

Housemate: 'You're full of energy today. Must be because you haven't gone to the gym.'

Oh crap, she's noticed I haven't gone.

She must think I've put on a shit load of weight.

Why else would she make that comment?

On the way to the shop.

Housemate: 'It's good to see you more often and with energy.'

What's her motive here?

Absolutely petrified that she thinks I'm fat, I decide to take a risk and change my routine.

Change from going to the gym as soon as it opens, to going sometime in the day.

By going I'll still be exerting control over my body, and the energy I'll save by not waking up early to go can be invested into my relationships with others.

Or not.

It's ten in the morning, so not necessarily peak time, yet the gym is rammed.

Rammed with people skinner than me, pushing harder than me, going faster than me, lifting more than I can.

Even before I go on the first machine a battle ensures in my head.

One voice tells me that I am inferior and that I shouldn't be seen in here. I'm an embarrassment after all.

The other voice tells me not to let what I see defeat me.

That in time I'll be able to match them. In fact, with a little bit more time, I'll surpass what they can do.

With no chance of being able to go back to Kent and get the inpatient treatment I desperately want and need, I decide to listen to the latter voice and keep going with it. After all, stopping going to the gym coupled with an inability to stop eating means that I will be the size of a horse in no time. And all that effort to be accepted will be for nothing.

So I force myself back to the gym.

At a reasonable time.

But I can't shake the feeling of utter self-revulsion.

At my body.

So I cover up. From head to toe.

Refuse to remove any layers. Even when I overheat

I'm also on high alert.

Alert to any movement in my immediate vicinity.

Giving death stares to those who not only dare use a machine next to me, but those who proceed to perform better on it than me.

Niggling voice: *'Holly you are being rude to others. You know what that means.'*

Yes.

Punishment.

With a heavy heart, I stop going to the gym.

That's not enough.

I quit the surfing and athletics club (not that I've been because you know, too fat to go in the first place).

Still not enough.

So I start forcing myself to eat more.

Punishing myself by doing the very thing I don't want to.

I eat two gigantic salad sandwiches a day.

This is soon accompanied by fruit.

One banana with each sandwich.

One soon turns to two bananas, three bananas, four, five, six bananas.

Now comes the smoothies.

One a day, two a day.

Please, please, please, someone help me stop eating.

But nothing can stop it.

I sit in my bedroom shaking with every passing day.

Struggling to breathe.

Struggling to calm my mind.

I'm drowning in the grips of an addiction to eating.

It shouldn't be like this.

I shouldn't be eating at all, let-a-lone eating so much so soon after months of not letting any food pass my lips.

The thought comes back into my head.

This time much stronger and persistent.

The least I can do is give it a try.

So I move from my bed to the sink.

I tentatively stick two fingers in my mouth.

Nothing.

I slowly move my fingers deeper into my mouth.

Nothing.

I try again.

I gag.

I throw myself back onto my bed and cry.

I can't stop eating.

I can't make myself sick.

I can't exercise.

How can I show my face at the eating disorder service?

My desperation at not wanting to feel like this pushes me to go to the appointment.

There's no-one in the waiting room apart from the receptionist.

She chats to me about nothing in particular.

Looks at me like I'm just another person.

She makes me feel like I'm anywhere but where I am.

This is odd.

The therapist calls me in.

She's tall. Taller than me.

She has broad shoulders and is big boned but not fat.

I'm big boned.

She talks to me about food and eating.

I reply.

She nods and takes notes. I can't tell what she is thinking.

We finish.

Therapist: 'You have Bulimia Nervosa.'

But I'm not making myself sick

Therapist: 'We will offer you an eight-week group nutrition course and sixteen weeks of individual Cognitive Analytical Therapy. Both will start in a few months. '

She's challenging me. Seeing if I can make myself fit into the diagnosis. In a short amount of time.

The pressure consumes me.

⸺

Emotionless.

Numb.

Despondent.

I'm surrounded by bleakness. Stranded in the moment. Nothing positive to look back on and nothing in the future to focus on.

Doing what I need to do to survive, I go to see a student about being her weekend live-in carer.

Gerty: 'I'll also need you to cook and make meals.'

All of a sudden my mind is filled with horrifying images of cutting my stomach and slicing my neck open.

What if she expects me to eat too?

Oh G*d, oh G*d, oh G*d.

Deep breathes.

It'll just be a moment in time. You'll be paid to cook for her, not for yourself.

You need the money.

You need to be distracted.

Take it but don't commit to it.

So I take the job.

I take it without feeling. Hoping it will fill the void of nothingness.

But it doesn't. It simply grows and strengthens as the amount of time spent in my room waiting for Gerty to tell me what she wants and needs, increases.

I feel surplus to requirement.

Surplus as a carer.

Surplus to requirement as a friend.

Surplus as part of a family.

Surplus to requirement to be educated.

Simply surplus to requirement to life.

Unable to confront my unwarranted existence out of sheer fear, yet still clinging onto the thread of hope that things may change, I cut out everything I deem unnecessary.

Developing existing friendships and making new ones.

Goodbye.

Attending lectures.

No more.

Looking after my physical, mental and spiritual wellbeing.

Long gone.

Handing in coursework.

Just about.

Going to work.

Physically there, mentally elsewhere.

Eating.

Unwanted but unstoppable.

But there's one thing I can't shift.

That I've never been able to shift.

The crushing weight of letting others down.

Putting it off for long enough, I text Josh. Finally agreeing to meet up.

Accepting that I won't be able to not eat, I allow myself a banana.

Again, one, turns into two, which turns into three and finishes at four.

Four leads to excruciating stomach cramps.

Cramps that go just before we are due to meet.

Phew. I haven't let him down.

Niggling voice: *'Doesn't mean that he won't let you down.'*

The niggling voice is right.

As soon as we are in town, he points out girls who are much skinner than me.

Why is he doing this?

Maybe I deserve this?

No, I don't.

So I pick him up on it.

As pointless as that is.

He tells me that they are not too skinny. He tells me they are pretty.

He goes a step further.

He tells me I'm curvy.

A step too far.

What is wrong with him?

He doesn't get it. Like really doesn't get it.

Whilst still traumatised by his remark, he decides he needs to take pictures of me.

Not just one or two. Bordering on fifty!

Josh: 'Look up at me, look to the left, move your legs, go stand by the lighthouse, hands in pocket.'

Are you actually kidding me?

Why can't I say no?

What is he going to do with these pictures?

Holly: 'Can I see the pictures.'

He shows me.

But only one, or two.

I ask to hold the phone to get a better look.

He refuses.

I ask for him to send them all to me.

Again, he refuses. Says he will only send a couple.

What is he playing at?

I leave it. Too scared to think what the answer may be.

Instead, I focus on the fact that the person in the pictures is not as fat and disgusting as I feared.

The relief this brings makes me glad that I made the effort.

Not with Josh per se. He has annoyed me.

More the fact that I made an effort socially.

So I decide to carry on.

This time, with people I hardly know.

Not wanting to blur the lines but thinking they wouldn't keep asking me if they didn't want me to go, sees me relent and join Gerty and her friends at the Student Union quiz.

Go and be other-focused. You don't and shouldn't need to talk about yourself.

Holly: 'Yea, so I don't have a good relationship with food.'

What the hell?

Katie goes silent. Deadly silent.

Gerty: 'I assumed as much as you don't eat with me.'

Oh, fuck. How did she pick up on that? Will I lose my job? Will Katie talk to me again?

I retreat further inside myself praying for the night to end.

It comes.

Comes with the strangest ending.

They hug me.

What is this? Why are they hugging me? This is something the 'fake' girls do. Not me.

Nowhere near able to or wanting to process what just happened sees me throw it far into the recess of my mind where I hope it gets forgotten.

But instead of being forgotten, it starts to signify a change.

A change in my social world.

I start to spend every weekend and maybe once a week with Gerty, Katie, Jesse and Patricia.

I start going ice skating once a week with a coursemate.

I make more of an effort with my housemates and spend more time with Josh and Luke: a guy from the debate team I met the previous year.

I also meet Jasper. In a lecture.

Afraid to force something that may not be there as I did with Josh, makes me wary to carry on talking once the lecture finishes. However, seeing that like me, he doesn't know many people on the module, I have a change of heart.

So we chat, swap numbers, spend time outside of lectures together and are soon enough dating.

Things appear to be on an up.

Niggling voice: 'Not for long.'

Being in a relationship, I need a hot bod to suit.

Having friends, I need a hot bod to suit.

To do well academically, I need a hot bod to suit.

Going on holiday with Steven, I need a hot bod to suit.

I'm sure you get the picture.

If it's not enough to contend with having a fat body on holiday with a stick thin Steven, I have to deal with my body betraying me yet again.

Betraying me in the worst possible way and at the worst possible time.

Nine months without has made me feel so, so, so good. It gave me a much needed breather where I could prepare for its return. Replace the over-eating, binging, late night/early morning snacking and exercise withdrawal with what I wanted to do the first-time round. To love and care for my body through healthy eating, exercise and self-love.

Instead it comes back out of the blue in the middle of our holiday.

Being totally unprepared and not able to shake Steven, I'm left with no choice to tell him I need to go to the pharmacy.

Steven: 'What for.'

Oh for fuck sake Steven. Do you really have to ask?

Holly: 'Sanitary towels.'

I'm filled with utter shame and embarrassment.

Hours later my fingers are back down my throat.

What's this? Have I actually done it?

I look down.

Phlegm.

Laughable I know, but it's a start.

You've done it girl. As soon as you get back to Plymouth, go and buy yourself some more of those go-ahead yoghurt bars as a treat. Promise not to tell anyone!

So, upon my return, off I trot to the shop like a good girl.

Numerous voices run through my head.

Get the bars. Nothing bad will happen, after all you can all but make yourself sick. The bars can be your practice. You'll nail it in no time!

Don't get the bars, you don't need them. You don't need to make yourself sick. Get some fruit. Eat healthily.

Leave the shop now! Right now, without buying anything. You don't need food. Look at all the damage it has caused you since you started eating again. You don't need that kind of shit in your life.

Knowing that I don't have the willpower to stop eating again leaves me with two options.

So I pace the aisles picking items up and putting them back down again.

I'm physically and mentally going round in circles.

Reverting back to what I know, I look at calorie content. 71 calories per bar. Pretty much the same as a banana. If these are easier to bring back up then bananas, then they're going to be what I buy.

They fail me. They bloody well fail me. Why the fuck can't I make myself sick properly?

What are you going to do next?

No, surely not.

I see them in my mind's eye.

I walk over to my desk.

Pick them up.

Sit on my bed staring at them. Rolling them over in my hand. Envisaging what I'll do. How I'll do it. Where I'll do it. What it'll feel like.

In a trance I open them up. Stare at their sharp tips.

Place one tip on my arm.

Visualise moving them along my arm as quick as you would rip a plaster off.

All a sudden queasiness hits.

I throw the nail scissors across the room and storm out of the house.

Without realising it, I'm leaving the shop having bought two Fiji milkshakes.

The only compensation I can offer my mind is that these milkshakes will begin my return into full starvation as they have in the past.

I'm not okay with this thought. Really not okay with it. But with no choice, I return home locking myself in my room with the TV blaring as a means of distraction as I down the drinks I really don't want and definitely don't need.

I should off known by now that I'm unable to exert any self-control.

And with that comes dire ramifications.

Dire ramifications including no longer being able to zip up my size 8 skirt all the way up.

No longer getting my size 8 jeans past my thighs.

No longer being able to freely move my arms in my size 8 coat without feeling restricted.

It's sickening.

Sickening that I've become so grotesque.

Grotesque not only to myself but to others as well.

Jasper: 'Why don't you come running with me.'

I panic. Slightly by the realisation that I've screwed up another relationship, but more so by the fact that in a matter of weeks I'll be back home for Christmas.

Back home seeing family and friends I haven't seen in ages, who haven't seen me in ages.

Where the sheer amount of weight I've put on will be more of a shock to them than to those I see regularly.

I'm back in Kent.

Stares in my direction are given. Lots of them.

Though questions and conversations about my weight aren't asked, questions about what may off caused my issues are.

Mum: 'Did something happen to you? Were you abused?'

What the actual?

Message received loud and clear.

With nothing bad having happened to me and not going through any 'acceptable' trauma, means that the reasons behind my eating disorder are not valid.

Not that I know the reason.

The thought hits me.

Now that my weight has gone up I have to justify my actions.

But how can I do that when I don't know the reason.

How can I appease everyone when one reason will not fit all.

It's not like I'll get away with giving different responses to different people.

Left with no option, I make a hasty decision.

A decision that I hope will see me return back to my anorexic days.

The days where I wasn't asked for a reason.

I buy a treadmill and cross trainer.

With the plan of locking myself in my room exercising twenty four hours a day, seven days a week, until I am thin enough to be seen.

The equipment arrives on New Year's Day.

Giving me a week to get fit and lose weight before my

housemates return and an additional week on top of that before the nutrition course starts.

Oh my dear G*d.

I can't run for more than five minutes.

Seriously, what is going on?

Fuck, what am I going to do?

Unable to cope with the realisation that I won't be able to lose the necessary weight sees a new plan unfold.

The plan to spend the next two weeks sleeping. Only waking to exercise and if absolutely necessary eat.

Eating being one piece of fruit a day.

I will not leave the house.

In fact, I will not leave my room except for going to the toilet.

It's the first day of the nutrition course.

Pushing myself to go means that I ignore my failures in exercising, in stopping eating and in not being seen by anyone.

I sing songs and create elaborate stories in my head on my way to the session: anything that will distract me from what I am about to walk into.

Yup. As I thought. Stick insects galore.

Great.

Though to be fair there is one person bigger than me. But who cares about her. Skinny is where it's at.

What a Bitch.

Spilling out of my size 8 jeans (yea, back in them, just), and pissed off that people seem normal (nothing of what I am going through is normal), I devise a new plan. Over the seven week course I WILL starve myself and act out. I'm fed up of not being taken seriously. If it's shock and drama that they want, then that's what they'll get.

And they get it.

Preparing for my fourth individual therapy appointment later that morning, I start by walking at pace on the treadmill.

You're still too fat and unfit to run.

Not being enough, I try to make myself sick.

You're a failure.

Needing to go to the appointment but not like this sees the veil lift to what I got to do.

Five minutes left before I need to leave.

I grab my water and reach to the back of my drawer.

1

2

3

4

5

No more Holly. No more

I head out.

When will it take effect?

What will I feel?

Should I say something?

I'm fifteen minutes into my appointment.

Holly: 'I've taken some tablets.'

The therapist asks me to repeat.

Holly: 'I've taken some tablets.'

Therapist: 'When? How many.'

Holly: '5, less than an hour ago.'

She leaves the room.

Comes back with another therapist.

They ask me more questions.

They try to get me to understand that this isn't right.

There's nothing wrong with it. It hasn't affected me.

They tell me that although I've only taken five tablets which isn't enough to cause any damage, I need to go to the hospital to get checked out.

Firstly, five is a lot. For me, who is not used to taking tablets.

Secondly, I'm not going to the hospital.

They tell me they won't see me again if I don't go.

Blackmailing me now, are you?

Fine whatever.

I leave, determined not to go, but knowing they will check up on me.

I'm standing in the centre of town feeling beaten. The only thing I have to cling on to is about to be taken away from me.

Not wanting to do this on my own I call Josh.

In a heartbeat he is standing next to me.

That's weird. Why is he here for me?

We head to hospital where we wait.

And wait

And wait.

I start to think back.

Think back to Steven and mine Year 9 parents evening.

On our way there, Dad seeks out the prices of a new housing development in front of Mum.

She's acting placid but I can sense she is hurt.

To Steven having a go at Mum one afternoon after school for not getting the exact ingredients he needed for cooking class the next day.

Mum by the kitchen sink crying before retreating upstairs to her bedroom.

To Mum's two children and Dad's two children never getting on and finding myself blaming my own existence for it.

To going to Zante with a group of school friends in the summer before starting University and being called the 'Adams family' by the eighteen to thirty's holiday rep.

To becoming aware of the inevitable demise of our school friendship group on a holiday to Newquay the following summer.

To Josh refusing to buy me a valentines card because he doesn't believe in it

Feeling not worthy enough as a result.

All I want is to be part of something.

Something infallible.

Unbreakable.

A nurse comes for me.

I talk like a child: quietly, using simple words.

He takes my blood and tries to weigh me.

I initially refuse the latter, but with no choice we strike a deal. There is to be no sniggering, laughing, facial expressions or verbalising what the scales say.

I'm putting a lot of trust into him, he better not break it.

He doesn't. But I'm still not pleased with him. He had no right in forcing me to be weighed.

In fact I hate him right now. I absolutely, unequivocally hate his guts.

The failure that I am sees my results come back clear. As punishment, I'm left hanging around for a further four hours to see a psychologist. A five minute consultation results in leaving with an appointment to see him again in two weeks.

Within a week the appointment gets cancelled.

History repeats itself.

It's not rearranged.

Niggling voice: 'Next time, you'll take more tablets. But for now just go through the motions of life'

So I go to work at the weekends, see friends, attend some lectures and work on my dissertation.

I tell myself not to bother any more mental health services.

To be content in the help I am currently getting.

The Dr. calls me.

Asks me to come in.

It's okay to ask for more help seems she called me, right?

So I tell her that I still plan to take an overdose.

She refers me to the Home Treatment Team.

⊏⊐

Three day later I'm being seen.

Of course it happens to coincide with Dad coming down.

Nevertheless, I have hope.

Hope that things will change. Change for the better.

Yet, the fear of being crushed when I'm inevitably let down sees me push down any hope.

And, surprise, I am let down.

They are arrogant.

They mock my attempt at an overdose to my face.

They talk to each other in front of me clearly insinuating that they don't believe me.

They suggest that I'm doing it for attention.

Oh, fuck you.

I just don't have the energy anymore.

Time for attempt two.

But before that I need to speak to Jasper.

It's been over a week since we last spoke and way longer since we last saw each other.

So I know what is about to come.

Fuck his explanation that he has tried to help me overcome my difficulties with food.

If you define help as telling me to go running with you, then, okay.

That he doesn't know what else he can do.

Errr, try asking how I am and listening.

That he wants to focus on getting into the Navy next year so feels he is not in the right place to be in a relationship.

That might be valid, but the fact that you say it last, means it's an excuse.

Probably for the best that he doesn't have a clue about what's going on with me at the moment.

At least he has the guts to end it himself, even if it is over Facebook.

━━━

With no more fucks to give I start to …

Drink to oblivion (not when working)

Eat boxes upon boxes of go-ahead bars.

Start making myself sick properly (thanks to my trusted toothbrush).

Take a handful of drugs on nights out.

Cut (well pierce my skin with nail scissors).

At the same time I continue to …

Go to the majority of lectures.

Hand in all coursework on time and keep on track with my dissertation.

Work at the weekends.

Attend therapy.

Make friends.

Start seeing someone else. Alan.

Alan, a housemate of Noah, a guy from my course I meet on a night out.

I know what he wants.

Sex. Just sex.

Why not?

So I sneak into his house late at night, and sneak out a few hours later.

It's thrilling.

We continue to see each other. Having sex whenever we want it and how we want it.

It doesn't matter that sometimes I get naked and other times I leave the majority of my clothes on.

I feel no pressure to be anything or anyone but me.

It's freeing.

Yet part of me feels like a prostitute.

But I can't help loving it.

I love it so much that I seek out highs.

So I cut, starve and make myself sick.

Yet I also hate it, so I chastise myself by also cutting, binging, making myself sick, drinking and overdosing,

This isn't right.

It really isn't right.

I've got to seek help.

Trembling uncontrollably, I open the Dr's door, sit down and take a deep breathe.

Four hours later I'm sat in the same room with the same two mental health professionals at the Home Treatment Team who dismissed me a mere few months ago.

Not offering any support, I leave.

I'm at home, having binged, thrown up and taken an overdose.

I lay on my bed listening to sad songs on repeat.

Suddenly I feel my heart race.

I begin to panic.

I run to the bathroom to throw up again.

Within ten minutes I'm back in my room where I fall into a restless sleep.

CHAPTER 7

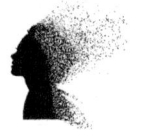

As tears stream down my face, I wonder if you realise the pain you're causing me.

I look out of my bedroom window searching for that one ray of light. I desperately reach out to it but end up stumbling forward as I see my hope my life, my glory being engulfed by you. I hear the rapturous laugh as the thunder bellows and lighting crashes all around me. Every shape and sound my mind conjures up reverberates like the poisonous words thrown as daggers towards me.

I have nowhere to look, nowhere to turn, nowhere to be.

You are now me as I am you.

Not only is everything coming to an end, I'm forced to mark them as such.

Writing goodbye letters in therapy.

Sitting final exams at University.

Going to the summer ball with friends.

Soon enough I'd be saying goodbye to Alan.

I can't have it end. Not like this.

Education.

The one thing that has always been important to me.

Knowing that it's unlikely I'll get a good grade, I spend hours looking for post-graduate courses that will accept me.

There's two.

I apply for both.

I get an unconditional offer from one and a conditional offer from the other.

Of course the conditional offer is the one I want.

So I work hard.

Bloody hard.

But it's not enough.

Not taking it lying down, I fight and get extenuating circumstances from the University.

They tell me that I can either re-sit my exams in the summer or repeat the year.

Fuck repeating the year AGAIN.

Choosing to re-sit, I email the MSc course administer pleading my case and arrange to stay living in my room for the rest of the summer.

I really don't want to go back home.

———

Out of the blue I get an email from Bournemouth University.

I've been accepted onto the course. With my grades as they are.

Fuck re-sitting the exams.

So I don't.

But I resubmit my dissertation.

Crap.

I need a place to live.

Crap.

I have no money until I get the career development loan.

Which I won't get until I confirm my place on the course.

Olivia who has moved into the house for the summer, and who, as it so happens, is transferring to Bournemouth University in September, offers to lend me the deposit.

If we live together.

Alarm bells ring.

Fuck it. I need somewhere to live.

Things are looking up.

More so when Alan moves in for the summer.

Well this could be fun.

Niggling voice: 'So you think.'

Straight away Olivia tells me that she is more suited to Alan.

Despite her having a boyfriend.

A boyfriend that she will likely cheat on. As she likes to tell me she has with all her previous ex's.

Those alarm bells were ringing for a reason.

I speak to Alan.

He doesn't give two figs. In fact he quite likes the fact someone is interested in him. So much so that I catch her in his room late at night talking.

They tell me time and again that nothing is going on. Yet they continue to flirt right in front of me.

I thought with Alan moving in, we would be having a lot more sex. But no, it's had the opposite effect.

That's because he prefers Olivia to you.

She's much more outgoing, flirtatious, sexual and sensual than you.

You're a plain Jane.

I need a fresh start.

Bournemouth is offering me that.

But I can only do it with Olivia's financial help.

So I suck it up.

I let her and Alan flirt away. Let them continue to meet up in his room late at night.

It's not like we are going out or anything. And as soon as I move to Bournemouth we will be over.

CHAPTER 8

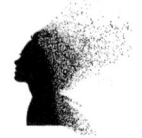

AND WE ARE OVER.

I decide to chalk it up to experience.

I also chalk up everything else my last year in Plymouth threw at me to experience.

Experience that has no place in my present or future.

Yet it continues to infiltrate everything.

IT'S our first week in Bournemouth. Olivia decides to stock up on food.

A new housemate arrives.

Housemate: 'That's a lot of food you both have.'

IT'S NOT MINE!!

Don't say that. You can't say that.

*Oh G*d, he thinks I'm a pig.*

I implore Olivia to tell him it's all hers.

She does.

He still laughs about it. Doesn't believe it.

Fuck.

It's because I'm fat. There's no way in hell he would make that assumption if I was skinny. If I were the size I was last September.

Okay Holly, it's just one situation. Olivia told him the truth. Give her the benefit of doubt.

She may not be out to get you.

Olivia comments on the nice figure I have. That I should wear clothes that show it off.

I don't understand why she is saying this.

Is she trying to make up for her actions in Plymouth?

Is she trying to come on to me?

Is she trying to fool me into wearing something that makes me look grotesque?

I decide to give it a go.

So I wear my long white summer skirt and a red top.

We go for a walk in the park.

Olivia: 'That guy is checking you out.'

Is he hell.

You're saying that to tear me away from Alan!

Later in the walk…

Holly: 'I don't like the back of my knees.'

Olivia: 'Oh don't worry, I know slim people who have a lot of fat there.'

She's calling me fat!!

We also talk about Plymouth.

Olivia: 'I've been talking to Alan.'

You what?

Holly: 'How are you talking to him?'

Olivia: 'We swapped numbers.'

Excuse me? You swapped numbers without me knowing.

Knowing that it would hurt me.

Olivia: 'He is really flirty isn't he?'

Oh for crying out loud. You can talk!

Her flirtations knows no bounds.

Steven comes down with his boyfriend.

Olivia: 'He is so good looking. It's a shame he is gay. I bet I can turn him.'

Seriously? You think that much of yourself? And that little of Steven?

Her flirting only adds to Steven's dislike of her.

So he doesn't invite her to the pub with his group of friends who are also down for the weekend.

Tells me it's up to me if I invite her.

I do. Because I feel guilty.

Guilty and sorry for her.

━━━

IT'S PLYMOUTH GRADUATION.

It's meant to be a time of celebration.

But all I can focus on is it marking one year since I returned to University whilst anorexic.

More than that. How that one year has seen my weight balloon. More than double.

How am I supposed to stand there, walk on the stage, collect my certificate, have people applaud me, when I look like a whale?

Nevertheless, I go.

I go and tell myself that I've got this.

I tell myself to focus on what I've achieved, That despite everything, I've made it this far.

That Mum, Dad and Steven are here with me. Perhaps because they care? That even if I don't enjoy it now, it is something I can look back on fondly.

I make it through the ceremony.

Now to make it through the meal.

A meal I don't want. But feel pressure to have.

A meal where at any moment my friends could turn up.

Turn up and see me eat.

Oh G*d, they better not turn up.

Of course they do.

They turn up right before the food arrives.

Refuse to eat Holly, refuse to eat.

But I can't. Not in front of my parents and Steven.

So I eat. Feeling the anger rising with every bite.

Shortly afterwards Mum and Dad make their excuses and go back to the hotel. Steven heads to the train station.

I'm left with my friends.

My so called friends who forced me to eat in front of them.

I call an early night.

Arrange to see them tomorrow.

Needing to let lose, I text Alan again.

Of course he doesn't reply.

Fuck him.

Fuck Plymouth.

I'm ready to leave Plymouth for good and start afresh.

Gerty: 'My weekend carer hasn't replied to me yet. Can you stay this weekend and help.'

Holly: 'Sure. I can come down every weekend if you need me'

I'm obviously not ready to cut ties yet.

CHAPTER 9

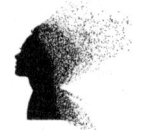

Haunted by thoughts of inadequacy, the heavily fastened doors gain an extra lock to its frame. Omitting the associated anguish these convictions hold by reinforcing their alliance with immoral people, allows you to grow with credence. Lost in copious amounts of shame, a snippet of anger is released through self-damage.
The induced high gets knocked of its podium from the accompanying low. Riddled with guilt I dissociate, flying far away from your antagonistic presence. The repetition of crashing down when reality draws me back finally boils over resulting in an explosion of years of pent up anger simply wanting to be accepted.

⸻

I know I don't fit into any eating disorder criteria.

I know that. I really do.

But I'm not right. Really not right.

I don't know what is going on. But I know that I need to take action to prove that something is going on.

To get help. Proper help.

This time I will speak up. I will tell the truth.

Will they see my truth as a problem worthy off treatment?

Is that a risk I can take?

Almost out of anti-depressants, I go to the Dr's for more.

Use this opportunity to ask to be referred for psychological treatment.

I'm given details of the University's Counsellors. One of whom is a clinical psychologist.

This could be promising.

I make an appointment.

That makes me feel good.

So I buy another ready meal. This time with a tub of ice cream and a big bar of chocolate.

Really Holly?

Knowing that I need to do all I can to be taken seriously, I put in action a new food plan.

Breakfast: nothing.

Lunch: swap coke for squash

Dinner: Ready meal.

Compensatory behaviours: make myself sick after eating.

It's an easy plan to follow. But it's not enough to stop the voice in my head.

You're not ill Holly.

There's nothing wrong with you.

You are a big fat fraud.

The voice continues to ring in my ears as I wait to be called in to see the psychologist.

Fearing I won't be believed, I exaggerate my difficulties as much as I think I can get away with.

Can't even stick to my promise to tell the truth. The whole truth. Nothing but the truth!

Why is he sitting so comfortably?

Why is he relaxed?

Why is he staring at me so intently?

Oh G*d. He must of sussed me out.

If I dare listen closely, I bet I can hear him laughing to himself about this pathetic excuse of a human in front of him, talking a load of crap.

So I shut up and wait.

Wait for the inevitable that he'll pass my case over to a counsellor. Someone less trained than him: less qualified. As, you know, I'm not severe enough.

He speaks.

He says he will work with me. That if I continue to make myself sick or begin starving again, he will refer me to the eating disorder service.

I should be glad. Happy in fact. But I'm not.

I'm not because I don't think I'll ever qualify for eating disorder treatment again.

Which means I am stuck with him. And I can't see myself working with him. There's just something about him I am not comfortable with.

What am I going to do?

CHAPTER 10

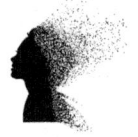

"Ungrateful, spoilt, attention-seeking Bitch"
come hurtling towards me like a moth to a
flame. My already beaten down soul
involuntarily welcomes the accolade.
Comparable to a bees need for honey is the
nauseous toxic taste your words bring. You
may sit there with a smirk upon your face,
but I sit there with anger seeping through my
veins.

I pause temporarily, my blurry vision taking
in the damage you've caused. The shock you
first ignited in me is now no more than a
sullen acceptance. Resembling a tattoo
fanatic, are the extensive sporadic and
meaningful cuts engraved in my arm. My
repeatedly inscribed initials are constant
reminders of the worthless failure that I
am. Only the sight of blood glistening off
my beloved 5 inch nail scissors fills me with

elation. Minutes of built up unbearable and disgraceful emotions finally run free.

◻▭◻

I need distracting.

So I put myself forward and get offered to work with the course programme director on his research.

Instead of giving me breathing space, it makes me want to self-destruct even more.

Now apt at making myself sick after eating, I decide to extent this to making myself sick after drinking. Not just alcohol, but coke, squash, water. Any liquid.

Easy.

Okay, next challenge.

Stopping food, or a large amount of food getting into my system in the first place.

Needing a deterrent, I chose cutting. The weapon of choice being scissors. My beloved nail scissors.

Facing my destiny head on, I sit on my bed with my left arm stretched out palm up and the nail scissors in my right hand.

I place the tip of one of the blades on my left arm, squeeze my eyes shut and slowly pull the scissors along.

Push past the stomach churning.

Start easy and slow.

You can miss your veins for now. As long as you draw blood.

Practice makes perfect.

Each tear of skin separating as the scissors move along my arm reverberates like a gun shot through my whole body.

I fling the scissors to the other side of my bed and look down at the damage I have caused.

I'm confused at what I'm seeing not equating to what I felt doing it. How can something that physically felt painful produce nothing more than a light scratch on my arm?

I haven't even produced any blood.

My insides are boiling.

I reach across the bed for the scissors and score my arm in the same place again and again.

The movement becomes more swifter the more annoyed I am getting at failing to produce any blood.

Attempt 2 – nothing.

Attempt 3 – nothing

Attempt 4 – still nothing

Attempt 8 – a trickle of blood appears on my arm and starts to pool.

I take a deep breath and sigh in relief. I let go of the scissors and slide down on my bed enjoying the feel of the throbbing cut.

I continue to cut.

Daily.

I also continue to restrict eating to the evenings. At a time when no-one is around and where I have free access to the bathroom.

With a routine set in stone, Olivia's pleads to join her and her new boyfriend for a night out in the pub becomes catastrophic.

Think Holly think.

Holly: 'I have no money.'

Olivia: 'We'll pay for you.'

Holly: 'I've got work to do.'

Olivia: 'It's only for a few hours.'

Fuck, what can I say now.

Out of excuses I reluctantly agree.

Holly: 'Okay, for one.'

I can substitute a night away from my routine if it means that I get to meet her new bloke and big him up to her to further ensure she has no reason to go back to Plymouth. Therefore, no reason to see Alan.

You can do this Holly.

With every drink I have I feel the shackles loosening.

Half way through the night it dawns on me that I can get a Chinese on the way home. I'd only be delaying my routine rather than forfeiting it. I'll just make sure that I shove that toothbrush right down my throat afterwards.

But how am I going to get away with this seems I said I have no money?

I know, I'll leave on my own. Buy the food. Scoff it in my room and then make myself sick all before anyone returns and without anyone knowing.

Ten minutes before the Chinese shuts, I make my excuses.

Of course Olivia insists on leaving with me.

For fuck sake!

I say I found a fiver and will get a Chinese on the way home.

Surprisingly she takes this fine.

So we leave the pub, go to the Chinese, head home, eat the food and then go to bed.

I do this all without making myself sick or cutting and not feeling bad about it.

That doesn't mean that I don't make myself sick the next day, or the day after that, or even the day after that.

Even knowing that the one toilet in the house is playing up and is likely to break, can't stop me from making myself sick.

I eat a prepackaged salad and throw up.

I see the sweetcorn and lettuce leaves swirling in the toilet.

Ten minutes later and sure that I've expelled everything, I flush the toilet praying that the evidence will go with it.

It doesn't work.

That's okay, it's taking a few attempts at the moment.

I wait for the pump to refill then try again.

And again. And again.

Nothing.

Feeling unphased, I'm left with two choices.

One – scoop the food up in a bag and dispose of it in the bin.

Two – just leave it and plead ignorant if asked.

Number one isn't an issue. I've done it before. But for some reason I decide on option two.

So I go to my room and wait.

There's a knock on my door.

Olivia: 'The toilet isn't working and there's food in there. Is that you.'

Holly: 'Nope.'

Vehemently denying it doesn't convince Olivia. Not that I could care less.

What I do care about and what I hadn't taken into consideration is that I won't be able to use the toilet to make myself sick. Not until it's fixed.

We can use the toilet in the self-contained flat attached to the house, but I can't use it to make myself sick.

Right Holly, you will cease eating until the weekends when you are at Plymouth and have access to your own toilet. Stick to cutting in the week.

Not sure whether I have the willpower to carry this through, makes me glad the second appointment with the counselling service is coming up.

Explaining how I've been making myself sick after every

meal, upped the self-harm and my attempt to explain the internal battle in my mind, leads to nothing other than my next appointment being booked.

Turns out his promise of referring me on was a lie.

Apparently I can be fooled once, twice, three times and forever.

As usual, I carry on. I go through the motions. With no enjoyment.

Attend lectures

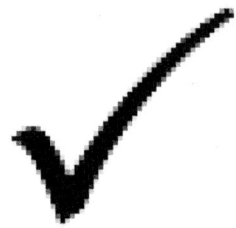

Hand in coursework and sit exams

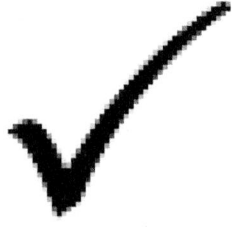

Work each weekend down Plymouth

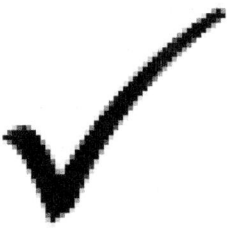

Volunteer as a research psychologist with the programme lead

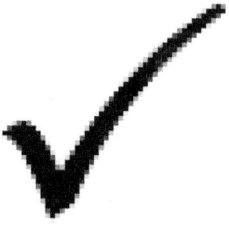

Get offered a clinical support worker job

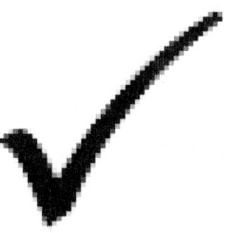

Make myself sick (now the toilet is fixed)

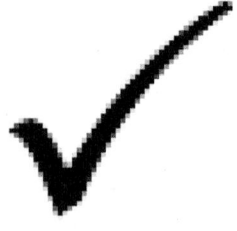

Cut

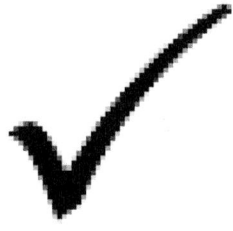

Speak to Alan

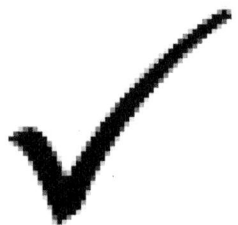

Speak to him despite weeks of radio silence.

Speak to him even though he bangs on about other girls he is interested in.

It's fine. It's not like we are together.

Speak to him despite knowing that he is only messaging me as him and Olivia hardly talk any more.

Still speak to him because he wants to start sexting.

Ha, me sexting? That's laughable.

The ever obliging person that I am, sees me agree to this.

He talks to me dirty.

I don't have a clue what to say back.

He sends me pictures. Asks for some back.

I attempt to take pictures of myself but am grossed out.

I don't send any back.

I tell him again that I'm down every weekend and am up for no-strings attached sex.

Five weekends later he agrees to meet.

Probably because he isn't getting anywhere with anyone else.

He'll meet only if I come to his in the middle of the night then leave straight away.

Wow, okay. Shameful.

Wanting to be wanted, I do it.

Thirty minutes after sneaking in, I sneak out. Feeling numb but with no regrets.

At least I'm wanted.

———

So, Friday to Mondays are taken up with working in Plymouth, spending time with friends and the potential of seeing Alan.

Wednesday and Thursday are spent in lectures.

Tuesdays is my homework and research day.

Each day is also for making myself sick and cutting.

Having a routine gives me great comfort.

A routine that allows me to self-punish whilst also functioning makes me feel blessed.

Even more blessed by granting myself permission to up the harm when I'm feeling particularly anxious.

And I am getting more anxious. Anxious that we have a lecture on eating disorders by the person who runs the service.

Not having missed a lecture yet, and unwilling to do so sees me cut the deepest I have yet in order to calm my nerves. Calm me by its constant throbbing.

The lecture enthrals me. So much so that I find myself standing in front of the guy at lunch spilling my sorry story to him and asking for advice.

Without hesitation he tells me to go to my GP and say that he suggests I get referred to the eating disorder service straight away.

Wow.

I go. The GP is in a foul mood and is reluctant to make the referral, but does anyway.

You're a time waster. A strain on NHS resources.

I go home where I force myself to bring up all the fluid I had that day, to self-harm then spend the evening in and out of crying episodes.

⸻

My behaviour starts to get more erratic as my thoughts become more distorted.

Once again I'm consumed by ripping the kitchen apart, screaming blue murder to everyone and anyone who dare cross my path, to start slicing my stomach and neck wide open.

At times I find myself hysterically giggling at these thoughts. Often at the most inappropriate moments.

I flee lectures with my toothbrush and nail scissors that I carry everywhere with me up my sleeve and head to the toilets.

I slam the cubicle door shut, sometimes not able to wait until the toilets are empty before I start forcing the toothbrush down my throat and start ripping my skin open. Not that I ever achieve more than a standard cut.

Nevertheless smirks rise on my face, making me bite my checks hard to supress them.

Though nervous at seeing the Dr again in case he is in a foul mood, I smirk as soon as he tells me I should hear from the eating disorder service in the next few weeks.

Bite your checks. HARDER.

Failing, I talk with my head hanging down thinking of what else I can do to make myself skinner and quick smart.

Laxatives – that didn't work last year. Plus I don't want to sit on a loo all day and night, especially as our toilet is liable to breaking.

Starving – been a year and a half since I started eating again and hundreds of failed attempts to stop again. So that's not going to happen.

Over exercising – haven't even stepped foot in the gym so that's also not going to happen.

Making myself sick – already doing that. Maybe I can do it more?

Being my only option, that's what I got to do. That and continuing to self-harm.

So I do, even though sometimes I don't want too.

Shush, that's a secret not to be spoken of.

Ever.

Before I have chance to blink, an appointment with the eating disorder service comes through. An appointment in less than a week.

Pressure much!

With my spiel on point, I go in somewhat confident that I'd be able to get support from her.

So it comes as a shock when she begins interjecting and probing everything I say: often stopping me mid-sentence.

Yea, I know that's her job.

It is also a shock when she sums me up all but perfectly at the end of the session. Stating that I respond with factual knowledge rather than from an emotional perspective.

Surely that means I don't qualify for treatment.

But she offers to work with me. For sixteen weeks. Using the treatment of choice: Cognitive Behaviour Therapy (CBT).

I'm suddenly on a high.

A big high. That lasts for a good five seconds.

Frankie: ' Go buy this book which we will be working from.'

Huh? A book? A self-help book? You got to be kidding me. This is not CBT. Anyway, self-help books are a pile of crap. Written by people wanting to earn money from those who are vulnerable.

I leave the appointment. Thinking.

Could I be wrong about the use of a book in treatment?

Do I not know as much about CBT as I think I do?

Well obviously not. She's qualified, you're not.

Not being the outcome I want, I tell myself to forget the treatment. To carry on being ill. To finish my Masters, return back home skinner than before and ask to get admitted to the Kent eating disorder service.

They haven't contacted you yet so you're still in with a shot of getting back in there.

Seven months until you can return home is nothing.

You can do this.

No. Wait a minute. Give it a go.

Use your treatment at Plymouth and Bournemouth as evidence that outpatient treatment isn't enough.

So I order the book and read the first couple of chapters before my next appointment.

At the same time I continue to self-destruct.

Not just through cutting and making myself sick, but also through alcohol.

I've never been much of a drinker.

Not much a fan of the taste.

Only drink because that is what you do as a teenager and whilst at University.

More than happy to stop. But it offers protection. Protection from thinking and acting like the social inept being that I am.

So when I'm out with friends I drink.

Sometimes it works.

Sometimes it doesn't.

Most of the time it makes me feel utter self-contempt.

Whatever the mindset alcohol brings, it numbs me. Numbs me enough to allow me to cut.

Cut deeper.

Stops my gag reflex so I can be sick as much and as often as my heart desires.

Alcohol has always been used as a way to function not only in an acceptable way, but in a way that would draw people towards me.

18th birthday surprise:

Gemma had organised a surprise birthday meal at TGI in London for Steven and I for our 18th after school. I could label the shock I felt at someone doing this for us and people wanting to come, but I couldn't label all the other emotions swirling around my mind and body. So I drank and acted more drunk than I was after the meal and on the train home.

School friends 18 birthday party:

Still part of the 'popular' group at school, but having gravitated to our group in recent months, a friend invited us to her joint 18th birthday party with another 'popular' girl.

Surprisingly confident in going, it wasn't until I was there that I was filled with great anxiety. Despite the shallowness and immaturity of others that I knew I didn't want to be part of, I felt my hand was forced in drinking from being in a situation I didn't feel I fitted into.

University of Plymouth Badminton social:

With drinking being at the core of all sport socials, I knew what the night would entail. But what I didn't expect was to feel so crap about myself. Moving from the student union to a club we played a drinking game where a girl would lie on the pool table with a full shot glass in her mouth. A guy would then volunteer to take it from her using his mouth. After much deliberating I put myself forward. At the exact moment a guy stepped forward, everyone's attention was drawn to the clubs photographer taking pictures. As soon as the picture was taken, everyone separated leaving me lying on the table like an idiot.

A very unattractive idiot.

My all-encompassing need to self-destruct begins to infiltrate my dreams.

With the increasing deterioration of my mental state not being taken seriously I feign fainting episodes in various locations when someone is walking past. As a result I am hospitalised where I undergo numerous tests.

Of course, tests that could offer a physical explanation.

Finding nothing I'm discharged.

A couple days later I 'faint' again, being re-hospitalised and having more tests done before being discharged.

Faint, hospitalised, tests, discharged. The cycle continues.

That is until the Dr's become savvy.

Needing to be seen, to be noticed, I starve myself dropping to four stone with only a few weeks left to live.

Finally I'm held under the mental health act, placed in isolation and am tube fed.

Doesn't matter that only Dad comes to see me. That the rest of my family have disowned me. I'm finally being taken seriously and getting the help that I need.

All of a sudden I'm jolted awake, in a cold sweat and struggling to catch my breath,

Night after night I'm plagued by this nightmare and each time it comes with increasing intensity.

Such intensity that I cannot shake it in the day.

It's all-consuming and all convincing that this is the thing I got to do next.

That I have no choice.

Oh G*d, oh G*d, oh G*d. What am I going to do?

In a bid to placid it, I think of situations and places that I can re-enact this. Hoping and praying that it will never come to fruition.

⊏⊐

All my efforts to try to push the nightmare down are thrown up in the air a few weeks into the new year when I get a phone-call from Kent eating disorder service.

Fuck. Couldn't they off waited another 6 months? When I've prepared my body and mind for it.

What the hell are they going to say?

What the hell am I going to say?

Therapist: 'We want to offer you to start outpatient treatment.'

Fuck. What can I say? Surely the truth will make them retract the offer.

Holly: 'Erm, err. I'm currently away doing my Masters .…. And am receiving support from their service.'

I hold my breathe.

Therapist: 'Okay. If you still need support when you return home then give us a call and we will see you straight away.'

And breathe.

Did that really happen?

Things are starting to look up.

More so when I find out I'm getting high 2:i's and 1st's in my coursework and in class tests.

Niggling voice: *'Don't worry, it'll come crashing down spectacularly.'*

Two half day lectures on personality disorders.

We talk about the three clusters.

We go through the personality disorders contained in each cluster.

Cluster A: paranoid, schizoid and schizotypal.

Okay, fine.

Cluster B: antisocial, histrionic, narcissistic, borderline.

Oh shit.

Borderline's are known for having:

Unstable self-image

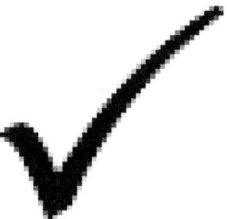

Recurrent suicidal behaviour or self-mutilating behaviour

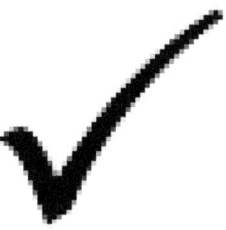

Chronic feelings of emptiness

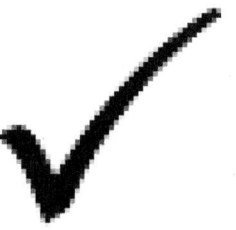

Abrupt shifts in mood

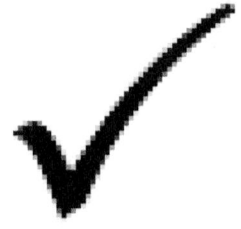

Fear of abandonment

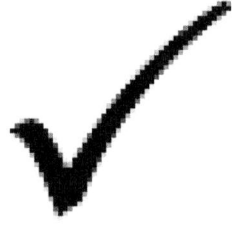

Unstable and intense interpersonal relationships

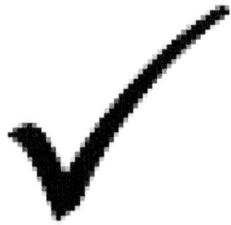

Feelings of disconnect from the world, own body, thoughts and behaviours

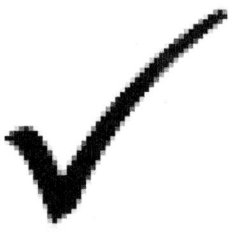

Inappropriate intense anger

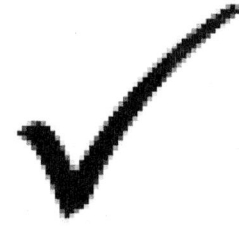

My head spins.

Nausea rises inside me.

The walls are closing in on me.

I struggle to catch my breath.

My whole body shakes.

I feel my face burning.

Unable to escape without drawing attention to myself, I zone out of the lesson and replay all the memories I have access to, to see if they fit the criteria.

⊏⊐

Steven and Julie fighting

Breaking up Steven and Julies constant verbal and physical fights.

Finding myself treading on eggshells to be on both of their sides without upsetting the other and without the other knowing. Coping with the feelings that I'm betraying both of them by detaching from the environment and from my body.

If I'm not (mentally there) then I can't be blamed.

Starting secondary school

Used to having Steven with me twenty four hours a day, seven days a week, saw me continue to rely on him at secondary school. That's until I made a new friend and I told him to piss off when he was hanging around me at lunch time.

You're a bitch Holly. Use him when you need him. Dump him when you don't.

My 12th birthday

A friend getting our form tutor and the rest of the class to sing happy birthday to me in the afternoon. My instant reaction of 'that's nice' was quickly replaced with 'why the hell did he have to do that. I hate his guts' all because he made me late for my favourite lesson.

Why can't anything ever go perfectly?

Mum's tape recording in my first year at Plymouth University

Mum sent me a tape recording after hearing that I'm not eating. I understood that it was out of love but I was still filled with anger and resentment. I could hear the underlying tones that I'm being stupid and an idiot.

Why on earth send a tape recording?

Obviously because she didn't want to come and see me. Say it to my face.

Doesn't want me anymore.

Stevens visit in my first year at Plymouth University

Steven and his boyfriend paid a surprise visit to me. Straight away my flat mates were on about how handsome he is, how it's a shame he is gay.

Hello, his twin is right here. I can hear you saying I'm the fat, disgusting one.

Why is he so perfect?

Why does he make me feel like this?

Why does everyone have to make it so obvious that I'm a monstrosity?

Weight comments

Working in a supermarket in the holidays, a colleague commented that I put on weight right in the middle of me buying my lunch.

Fuck you.

I'm going to stuff my face just to show you how unimportant you are to me.

My ex's step-mum comes into the shop a year later and bangs on about my weight loss and how it must have been University. All I wanted to do was to scream and shout at her that it was her step-son who has done all of this to me. That he has destroyed my life. That nothing is ever going to be the same again.

Why are people so blind to the truth?

Why does she have his back when my family don't have mine?

As soon as I get home, I'm straight on Google.

Eating disorders are common amongst people with borderline personality disorder (BPD)

Symptoms begin in teenage years or as a young adult.

The majority of people with BPD have been neglected or subjected to physical, sexual or emotional abuse during childhood.

Well that's not me.

I carry on reading.

BPD can also be caused by life problems when growing up, particularly in those who are naturally sensitive.

BPD has similar behaviour traits to autism.

People with BPD struggle to identify emotions and cannot express emotions appropriately.

It all makes sense.

I've grown up in a mixed and big family with a high prevalence of anxiety and Asperger's.

With so many of us, I never felt able to express my emotions therefore felt lost and misunderstood. As a sensitive child, I felt the only thing I could do was mould myself to be what people want me to be in any given situation, in any given moment.

So this is it.

This has been what's wrong with me for so many years.

It explains my constant need to self-destruct and why I cannot let go of my eating disorder.

Can't let go because I need it.

I need it to help me control and suppress my emotions. Particularly in situations that are unjust.

Needing to know for sure, I bring it up at my next appointment with Frankie.

I state the pattern of my behaviours.

From anorexia to bulimia to overdose to self-harm and their increasing intensity.

I talk about my constant self-hatred, black and white

thinking, impulsivity, sensitivity to environmental cues and identity disturbance.

I leave with a promise of a referral to the Consultant Psychiatrist at the eating disorder service.

From referral to an appointment within three weeks.

Twenty minutes into the appointment, BPD is confirmed with a prescription for mood stabilisers and a referral to the Intensive Psychological Therapy Service (IPTS) for in-depth assessment and treatment.

Be an adult about this, Holly.

So I let my family know. By text.

Hardly anyone replies. Because they don't care.

What more do I have to do to get them to show an ounce of care?

Nevertheless I feel liberated.

Liberated from knowing what is going on with me.

And liberated in no longer having to keep up a pretence of normal functioning.

So if I want to spend days starving myself of all food and drink, then I will.

Other days I may spend constantly cutting and taking overdoses.

Or I'll binge, either letting it stay in my stomach, or throwing it up afterwards.

I also feel free in telling and showing people how I really feel about them.

Never having gelled with her, I become short tempered with Olivia when I don't see the point in, or am not in the mood for talking.

I stand up to Alan, telling him that if he wants to have sex then he can come to me, rather than me always going to him.

I start listening to music in lectures, and presenting my work for marking with my hair all over the place, wearing baggy jumpers and no shoes.

I start smoking.

And I finally vent my frustrations about Katie to others. That she had drastically reduced what she eats, and steals my fags off me, denying it to my face.

Not only do I hate that she is copying me, I also hate that she is losing more weight than me.

So I decide to ensure that she eats more than me.

I agree to a dinner of Spaghetti Bolognese with friends.

I wait until Katie starts eating, mouthful after mouthful.

Then I push my plate away (having not eaten anything) and lock myself in my room.

Knowing that Katie now has more calories inside her than I do, tickles me.

Riding on a high, I take my nail scissors out from my bag and start cutting my arm over and over again.

Might as well do something proactive whilst everyone else is in the kitchen eating.

I continue being blunt and honest to others as well as destroying myself as much as I want to at any given time.

Until I start taking an overdose whilst I'm drunk.

At a weekend, when looking after Gerty.

With our friends over.

Realising what I'm doing, I immediately stop and text Hattie who is in the room next door, confessing my crime.

She takes the tablets and my drink away.

I promise that I will never do it again.

I feel such disappointment and disgust in myself.

How could I have done that to Gerty?

For the rest of that weekend and the following weekend I'm unable to look anybody in the eye.

Receiving an assessment pack from IPTS offers some relief.

Even though I know I will have to leave Bournemouth in five months if I'm unable to get a full time job.

Nevertheless I complete the questionnaires and attend the assessment appointment. To show willing.

They confirm that I have BPD.

They offer me Dialectical behaviour Therapy (DBT).

But the waiting list is 12 months.

Surprisingly all I feel is relief. Extreme relief that I have never felt with my eating disorder diagnoses.

Because I no longer have to fight for something. Something I didn't know I was fighting for.

With this, the shackles begin to loosen.

I reduce the times and intensity that I make myself sick and cut my arms.

I stop overdosing.

I start to see that people are not out to get me.

I no longer think that I have to be or act as I am the best in and at everything.

Nor do I need to control all situations.

So I genuinely sympathise with my course mates when they don't get offered an interview for the Doctorate in Clinical Psychology. And I celebrate when they get job offers.

I even swap my placement with a course mate as she really wants the one I was given.

I'm honest with the placement tutor in why I'm happy to swap.

Because I can't work at the service that has just diagnosed me with BPD.

He pulls me out of the placement. All the placements. My suitability to work with clinical populations is now being questioned.

He deems me to be too risky, He offers me to shadow a Consultant Clinical Psychologist in a mental health hospital.

By shadow, I mean sit in a room writing up my critical literature review and seeing him on two occasions for supervision and attending one multi-disciplinary meeting.

Not his fault. He is great. The placement tutor, not so much.

I read about the stigma associated with BPD.

I thought I'd be immune to it.

Yea, my family doesn't give two stuffs, but I thought that was just them.

Obviously not.

Might as well act as I'm being perceived.

So I let go of trying to function normally.

I let the severe self-hatred and delusions of grandeur come and go as they please.

Wanting to self-punish or knowing beyond any doubt that no harm will ever come to me, I continue to cut, overdose and either starve or binge followed by making myself sick.

Even in spite of knowing that having a routine can reduce my sensitivity to environmental cues, thus making me less likely to want to harm myself.

Yet, with Frankie's encouragement I try to stick to a routine, but it's hard. Particularly hard when I'm down in Plymouth each weekend, having no control over anything.

Even harder when I'm having to be social.

So much more harder when I know things are about to change for good.

But I try.

I force myself to go to Plymouth University Summer Ball with friends.

Despite having to wear my sisters dress as I can't find one that makes me feel the slightest bit okay.

Despite Katie looking super slim and being in a foul mood.

Despite Gerty wanting to call it an early night.

AND

Despite Gerty telling me that she found fags that she has stolen off me and some suspicious items in Katie's bag.

Are you bloody kidding me?

So, not only is she not eating much

Like me.

She is stealing things

From me.

G*d knows what else she is doing.

Not wanting anything to do with this and with Gerty having already sent Katie a text, I leave it.

CHAPTER 11

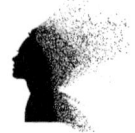

I HAVEN'T SECURED a full time job in Bournemouth.

I'm left with no option but to go home.

So I start to look for jobs in Kent.

I'm offered an interview a few weeks before I'm due to move back home.

So I pop back home for a few days for it.

I'm in the house on my own.

Thoughts of being a failure race through my mind.

I find myself in and out of the cutlery draws, testing the sharpness of the knives out on my wrists.

Then on my neck.

Running the blades back and forth.

Back and forth.

I imagine I am sawing a bit of wood in the backyard as I used to watch Dad do.

Slowly but steadily I begin to work my way through the layers of skin, fat (lots of it) and tissue.

I blink.

All of a sudden I am back in the present.

I find myself rocking to and fro by the kitchen sink with

various knives on the kitchen side and the sharpest one in my hand raised to my neck.

I quickly drop the knife to the floor and run to the mirror to assess the damage I have done.

I only see red and raised skin.

No blood and no tears of skin.

I sigh in relief, scramble back to the kitchen, put away all of the knives, leave the kitchen and the house. Going for a walk to clear my mind.

Not sure what to do, but knowing that I need help, I text Mum when I'm safely on the train back to Bournemouth.

I hope that it will spark concern and raise alarm bells.

It doesn't.

I get an angry text back.

I spend the rest of the train journey back crying.

I take one last risk.

I tell Frankie in our last appointment.

The offer is much clearer than the one from Kent.

Yet I refuse to stay in.

How can I take a bed in the unit being as fat as I am?

Telling her that I am moving home in a week and promise to keep myself safe is enough assurance for her to let me go.

Though part of me wishes she will force me to stay

So I leave.

I leave and go back to Kent. Moving back in with my parents.

CHAPTER 12

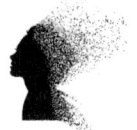

Erratic behaviour as a product of excessive
sensitivity to environmental cues engulfs
me.
Reactions are often and plentiful leaving my
body worn out and my mind in tatters. Each
thought, feeling and response is
idiosyncratic, leaving an unstable and
destructive path. Infinite causes maximising
their appearance hinders the ability to
manage robust emotions.

⊏——⊐

I would love nothing more than to smirk and stick two fingers
up at everybody who thought I wouldn't be able to get a job
after my Masters. And so soon.

But the job I have, as a carer in the community, is a job
anyone can get without any qualifications.

To rub salt into the wound, Laura has a similar job and my

friends girlfriend who didn't even go to University is in charge of assigning me clients.

Not that she treats me differently.

Though working with clients with mental and physical health difficulties gives me hands on clinical experience, I can't help but feel such a failure.

A failure who has wasted the last six years and has caused so much unnecessary stress on her family.

I've got to buck my ideas up. Quick smart.

So I call up Kent eating disorder service.

I tell them that I am now back in Kent and would like to take up outpatient treatment as offered.

The receptionist says she needs to check and get back to me.

Graham, the therapist calls back and offers me an appointment in just under two weeks.

I know I am a fraud as food is not the only, nor the main issue anymore. But I just don't have the energy to fight myself about this.

To figure out where the best place is for me and to try and get there.

So I take the opening.

But not without repercussions.

The repercussion of being compelled to make myself sick in order to at least partially fit in.

Living at home, I need to amend my technique.

So I only eat when expectations and eyes are on me.

I make my way upstairs at the end of meals when others are busy doing something else.

To reduce the noise in bringing the food up and from it hitting the toilet bowl and causing splash back, I slowly release the reproduced food bit by bit, whilst bending over the toilet as much as possible.

Aware that any length of time in the bathroom will arouse suspicion, I leave and return a couple of times within the space of half an hour.

Bringing up the majority of food the first time round reduces the separation anxiety from fear of having to space out my time in the bathroom.

I'm reluctant in telling my family that I'm back in treatment. Particularly after Mum's last reaction.

Yet, thinking it's better for them to hear it from me, I take the plunge.

Mum: 'Do what you got to do.'

Wow, she really doesn't care.

Rest of my family show no emotion.

I really am the worst person.

It makes me scared.

Scared and afraid.

Afraid as I know I'm a hotchpotch, in a hotchpotch family.

Born into and growing up in a tense and stressful environment.

Where, for whatever reason, I'm unable to safely and securely express myself.

Making me feel unloved, unwanted and not good enough.

Attempts at rectifying this as an adult with self-expression gets nothing but frustration from others back.

So I'm left to conclude that my life is pointless and I shouldn't exist.

The very thing that scares the bejesus out of me.

Unable to cope, I retreat further and further into my head.

Pulling me away from any meaningful interactions with others.

In no time at all I lose all confidence in speaking to anyone.

I question everything. When I'm meant to speak. How I'm

meant to speak. How I should respond. What my face should show and how my body should be.

I enter the eating disorder service. A thousand stone heavier than the last time I was there.

Please don't let me recognise anyone.

Please don't let anyone recognise me.

Receptionist: 'Hello.'

Fuck. What do I say. Hi. Hello. Alright. Hey. ???

Me: 'Err, Hi. I've got an appointment.'

She comments on my dress. The dress that I have deluded myself into thinking shows of my petite frame.

It's not until I get home after the appointment when I'm brave enough to fully look at what stares back at me in the mirror, that I see the true horror.

Thunder thighs.

The short hair highlighting the fatness of the face.

The unshapely and flabby old peoples arms.

Who is this person?

I feel physically sick that I didn't see this earlier.

How did I go in, confident in my ability to discuss my mental health history, particularly emphasising the eating disorder side of things.

I had no right to be there. To be seen. To talk freely and openly.

Oh G*D.

They didn't even weigh me.

Because I would of broken the scales.

Needing to quash these emotions RIGHT NOW, I gorge on a high carbohydrate dinner and chocolate pudding that disappears in mere seconds.

Torturing myself more, I go back to the full length mirror and stare.

Stubby legs with a huge amount of knee fat are reflected back.

The short sleeves of the dress emphasis the dangling fat hanging loosely from both upper arms.

Love handles that cannot be contained in the outfit.

Podgy cheeks and three chins accompany the four-eyed freak staring me down.

Where is the size six girl from two years ago?

Go throw up until there's nothing left. Then go and hide in your room.

You're an embarrassment.

An embarrassment that doesn't deserve to be seen.

To pay penance, I start slashing my arm.

Obviously, it's not enough. It never is.

I can't do anything right.

━━

Moving back to Kent, I really thought things would change for the better.

That living back with my parents and working would provide me with the structure and routine that I need to get my mental health back on track.

Instead I'm on a zero hour contract and am left to fend for myself.

Come and go as I please.

Cook and eat whenever and whatever I want.

Pick up as few or as many working hours as I can and I want to.

All that is needed of me is to pay my part of the bills and tidy up after myself.

All I want is to feel loved, that I'm making a difference and to have stability and consistency.

Dad taking me to my appointments helps.

Until Mum tells him not to.

That I have to do it on my own.

I get it.

But they don't get the importance of that emotional support.

Having a sporadic client caseload throughout the day and having to use public transport to get to their houses means a lot of wasted time and lack of planning and productivity in my spare time.

Not seeing my friends as regularly as I did during my placement year makes me feel isolated.

Hearing that Gerty won't be returning to University and that Katie is returning back to the UK after a month living abroad for her placement year makes me further question what the hell is going on.

Everything is changing.

And I have no control over it.

My existence is heavily pinned on others need and want of me.

That is hanging by a thread.

To take away this pain … to have some control … to feel cared for… I cut.

Deeper, harder and faster than before.

Not enough.

Knowing I care, but unable to care, I take an overdose. A couple of hours before I have a client that evening.

An overdose of more tablets than I've taken before.

I text my manager, say I've been sick and ask her to cover.

I sit on the sofa and wait.

I start to feel dizzy and sick.

I go to the kitchen and tell Mum I feel unwell and am going to bed.

I lie in bed convinced that this is it. My last night on earth.

I wait for God to come and take me.

Okay, not God, whoever it is that takes you to purgatory.

I battle to keep my eyes open as to prolong my life.

And I pray, despite knowing I shouldn't.

I wake up.

Dazed and confused I make my way downstairs for acknowledgement. To know that people see me. To hear them talk to me.

I know Laura is at work.

I hear Mum and Dad in their respective bedrooms.

I reach out touching various objects around the house.

I feel the fabric of the sofa, the hardness of the TV, the coolness of the fridge.

I open the window feeling the breeze upon my face.

I go out the back door and breathe in the fresh air.

So far everything points to me being alive.

But I don't feel alive.

I feel in no man's land.

Even seeing and talking to my parents is not enough to convince me of my existence.

Zigzagging others on the streets and helping clients makes me acknowledge that I still have a physical form, but not that I am still here.

I don't think I'll ever really be here again.

And I'm not.

I'm an empty shell.

I go to my weekly appointments at the eating disorder service: sitting there in silence, holding on tightly to the cushion on my lap and starring at the floor. He asks me questions. I either don't answer or give short replies.

But I tell him about my overdose.

He refers me to the Community Mental Health Team for a re-assessment of BPD.

It gets confirmed.

I'm put on another waiting list. This time, eighteen months.

Graham agrees to continue seeing me until I can start that treatment.

I tell Mum and Dad. They seem positive about the diagnosis.

What?

Can't and don't think I'll ever get my head around the sudden change in their reaction. Especially as the treatment will be three days a week between ten am and four pm for two years , meaning I will have to work part time, contribute less to the bills and be living with them for at least another three years.

Still numb, I continue to make myself sick.

Needing comfort, I go to see Mum in her bedroom after.

Mum: 'If you are going to make yourself sick, then there is no point in eating as you are wasting our food.'

I leave. Crawl into bed and curl up with my cuddly toys.

If I knew that's what she thought I wouldn't of tried so hard over the last few years to make myself eat when all I wanted to do was starve myself.

Now, it's too late. I no longer have the willpower to starve myself again.

Apparently I can no longer make myself sick. Not from the food at home.

Cutting and overdosing it is then.

They must get a thrill playing with my head. Toying with me.

Why else would they constantly have a go at everything associated with my mental health, yet want to celebrate events with me?

Not only do Mum and Dad come to my MSc graduation, so does Steven, Julie and her newborn son. They all stay the night. They all seem excited. They all seem (dare I say it) happy for me.

You're not the reason they have come down.

They just wanted to get away.

They are using your graduation as an excuse.

They don't care for you. Never have and never will.

Steven still wants to go on holiday with me over our birthday.

He tells me it's not a problem that at the last minute I decide I can't afford to go to France meaning that we will lose our non-refundable Eurostar train tickets.

He suggests we go to Edinburgh instead.

He subs me when I run out of spending money during the trip.

He says he is in no rush for me to pay him back.

Why is he being like this?

———

Something inside me is changing.

A sense of finality is washing over me. So strong that I feel powerless to stop it.

I'm becoming more drawn to the tablets. Not in taking them, but simply staring at them.

I'm also becoming drawn to my nail scissors. Laying them on the desk and sitting there, staring at them, contemplating.

Neither seem to hold much emotion over me.

Before, part of me would squirm at what I was going to do. Not now. They are simply instruments that will put me out of my misery.

They are nothing more, nor nothing less.

As the days roll by, my task becomes clearer.

I make one last attempt to reach out before the inevitable takes place.

I give our family Dr the letter I've written.

He calls the mental health team.

Can't get through.

Tells me he will try again later.

I leave, stopping at work before going home. Hand in my sick note.

I wait by my phone.

Nothing.

Needing to know I've done my all, I call the mental health team.

They haven't received a referral from my Dr.

I'm standing in the bathroom.

My phone rings.

It's Katie.

I pick up.

Tell her what I'm about to do then hang up.

I start inscribing my initials in my arms over and over again.

I watch the blood drip into the sink.

Drip, drip, drip, drip.

I take a concoction of anti-psychotics, anti-depressants and paracetamol.

I sit on the bathroom floor.

And wait.

One more try Holly. One more.

I reach for my phone.

Call 999.

I reply to Katie's texts saying an ambulance is on the way.

I head downstairs and wait.

Praying no one will come home.

Laura walks through the door and jokes that the ambulance is for me.

The paramedics come through the door.

I burst into tears.

I give them the tablet packages.

They make me give Laura my nail scissors.

I'm on the ambulance.

Laura is there.

I don't want her here.

I'm in A&E waiting room.

I start to feel dizzy and sick.

I'm on a trolley, refusing to wear the hospital gown.

I fall in and out of sleep.

Dad is there.

He calls me a stupid girl.

I tell him not now and turn over.

My bloods are taken.

They come back clear.

I'm ushered to another part of the hospital to see the mental health team.

I tell them in no uncertain terms that I want to be an inpatient.

They counter offer with daily visits from the home treatment team and support from a mental health social worker.

What choice do I have?

Forty-eight hours later I wake up in my own bed.

Dad tells me Graham has called as I missed an appointment.

Dad told Graham what happened.

He explained to Dad that I have serious issues.

You'd think that would be enough for my parents to be concerned about me.

Nope.

Mum, who has been giving me the silent treatment, storms into my room later that day, shouting at me and demanding answers.

In no uncertain terms I'm told that if I don't buck my ideas up right now I will be kicked out of the house.

Not knowing what to do, I hide out in my room.

I go on Facebook to seek solace.

I'm confronted with angry posts, from family, about the selfishness of suicide.

I read the numerous comments. All in agreement with them.

People know it's me.

I'm being attacked.

Gemma, Katie, Gerty and Hattie reach out to me.

I virtually cling on to them for dear life.

More so, when after three days, the Home Treatment Team discharge me. Just in time for Christmas.

Unable to be at home I spend Christmas with Gemma and the New Year with Gerty, Katie and Hattie.

Petrified that when I return home the locks would have been changed.

⊏▭⊐

Treading carefully not to rock the boat, I go to see the Dr on Mums say so.

As I am still in treatment and am waiting to hear from the social worker, there is not much he can do. Apart from prescribe me my medication weekly rather than monthly.

To reduce risk.

He also gives me another sick note.

With that in hand, I head to the office.

They know.

The whole office knows.

Julie has told them. Behind my back.

Who the hell does she think she is!

I'm seething.

Foaming at the mouth, unable to speak type of seething.

That's it. Fuck it. I'm taking up Gemma's offer and moving in with her.

But I can't.

If I move out, I can't come back.

Even though I strongly dislike my family right now, I don't want to risk losing them forever.

Plus it would mean stopping all treatment and having to, once again, fight to get my diagnosis reconfirmed and be put on more waiting lists.

So I stay put.

Lay low.

Ride out the storm.

It's not long until Thomas, the social worker calls ... offering a home visit ... offering to talk to my parents about what has been going on. To help them understand.

So I tentatively ask my parents if they would be okay with it.

They are.

How can they not be okay with me, but are okay with someone coming to talk about me?

Unless ... they think that this person is going to confirm their thoughts of what a bad person I am.

More evidence for them ... more ammunition to kick me out.

With the clock ticking down to Thomas's imminent arrival, I start pacing my bedroom floor with fear of what may be said.

He arrives.

Mum: 'Does she have Munchausen's?'

You what?

Surprisingly and immensely satisfying, Thomas explains BPD, linking it to examples of my behaviour and thoughts as well as connecting it with eating disorders.

More than that, he is not only able to explain, but also convince my parents that none of this is my fault and I am certainly not doing it for attention.

Just like that, they accept it for what it is.

More confused than ever (which is saying something), I retreat to my room as soon as Thomas leaves.

———

I am relieved. Very much relieved.

Relieved to the point that I want to stop acting like this.

Which I can, because my parents now believe me.

Right?

Wrong!

Reality hits.

Just because I feel accepted, it doesn't mean that I will automatically get better. I've got to fight to get better.

That means arming myself with knowledge about BPD and stating my case for intensive treatment at my appointment with the psychotherapist from the personality disorder service.

It works. My place gets confirmed. Just need to wait for a space.

If that's not enough, Mum shows interest. She asks me

questions. She researches BPD and the treatment I've been offered.

Graham also appears pleased that I've been accepted. He restates that he will still work with me until that treatment begins.

CHAPTER 13

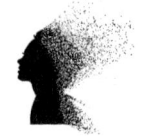

WHY ARE YOU ASKING?

It's Easter, not our birthday.

What are you planning?

Is this your idea or others?

You know I don't have much money.

You know I'm in debt.

Yet, you also know that I won't be able to say no to you.

You're planning on getting rid of me aren't you?

You want me to be complicit in it. That's why you are forcing me to organise it.

You suggest visiting two places. The aim is that the first place will make me think that we are on a 'normal' holiday, leaving the second place to be where you enact your plan.

Your plan to 'accidentally' lose me.

With my hands tied behind my back, I have no choice but to go along with it.

What will be will be.

Facing it like I would my own execution, I make the most of the first trip to Pisa.

Though unlikely to cause him any pain, as soon as we arrive in Florence, I try to keep my distance from Steven.

Making it easier on him to lose me.

I hide behind columns and wonder off on my own.

Steven gets annoyed at me. I can't understand why. I'm helping him.

I keep helping him, yet he always comes and finds me.

Before I know it we are on the plane back home.

What will my parents say when I turn up.

Will they blame Steven for not doing his job?

Will they disown him?

Do I need to disappear on my own accord?

What do I do now?

Carry on as normal, keeping an eye out for Steven, making sure no harm comes to him.

CHAPTER 14

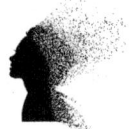

Feeling worthless from a young age I sought
to validate myself through the only means
available to me - education.
Success, Triumph, Accomplishment and Victory
became synonyms that are entrenched into my
psyche. Constantly aware of the need to
impress for acknowledgment, every effort was
made to be the best. Full concentration in
lessons and hours of extra circular work
proved futile. Failing to acquire invitation
to Mensa deduced my insignificance.

Ideas of grandiose develop in keeping of my
colossal need to make a difference in this
world. My talent having gone unnoticed
throughout school would resolve itself in
career aspiration from my tenacious mindset.

So I face my only survival mechanism bright

> eyed and bushy tailed, closing the door on
> anybody trying to reach me.

An act of carrying on normally is continuing applying for jobs.

With education and career success being everything to me, sees hope return.

Despite the numerous rejections I find sitting in my inbox.

Widening my net, I apply for jobs outside the elusive clinical supervision.

I also apply for a Doctorate in Counselling Psychology.

I get offered a job as a mental health recovery worker.

I also get an interview and placed on the reserve list for the doctorate.

With things looking up, I take the plunge and talk in therapy.

Not just talk about any old thing. Talk about something close to my heart. Something that I am rubbish at.

Relationships.

I start talking about Alan. How I had to accept his terms if I wanted to be with him.

The conflict these terms cause me as they go against my moral compass, yet they seem to be the norm.

The norm of what two consenting adults do. Particularly in situations such as being at University.

I find myself realising that it's not only the attention from him that drew me to him, it was also my perceived normality of the situation.

My need to be liked, wanted and accepted sees me go for guys where I feel I either have the upper hand (Josh) where I can control the situation, or where I become the vulnerable one (Alan), where I bend myself backwards to be what is needed. My fear of not being good enough therefore being abandoned, makes it hard for me to put an end to this pattern.

The insight gained from this session scares me.

Scares me because I realise how insecure I am. How reliant I am on other people. How I have no sense of self. How vulnerable I am.

So I shut down once again.

Go back to sitting opposite Graham, cushion held tightly over my lap, looking down and praying for the session to be over.

Also go back in repeating the same behaviour.

This time with Gemma's course mate.

Celebrating Gemmas birthday, I see her course mate staring at me.

All night.

Not talking to me, just starring.

When people leave, he stays.

He finally plucks up the courage to talk.

We chat.

Nothing more, nothing less.

He lingers.

We try to get him to go.

But he continues to stare and talk to me at the front door.

Everyone else disappears upstairs.

Great.

It's obvious that he wants to kiss me, but I just want him to go.

It's taking too long.

Thinking the only way I can get rid of him is to kiss him, sees me do it.

But he still stays.

Seriously?

Eventually I tell him I'm going to bed. On my own.

He leaves.

Finally.

He keeps texting.

I reply.

I agree for him to come down to see me.

But he has to stay at a hotel.

I have no plans to stay with him.

But I do.

I have no plans to sleep with him.

But I do.

He leaves the next day.

Relief washes over me.

I've given him what he wants, now hopefully he'll leave me alone.

Time to focus on the present.

All my siblings are speaking to me again. There's still tension but give it time.

Mum seems more accepting of me and my mental health.

I'm about to start a new job that is in keeping with what I've been studying.

Take it one day at a time.

So I try to push past the ever present thought that it has only been eight months since my last and most significant attempt at ending my life.

And the associated thought that this action, as a byproduct of my mental health, means that I qualify as a resident of where I am about to work.

Not letting this consume me, I start my new job with a big smile slapped across my face and willingness to work hard and learn fast.

To get the right balance where residents engage with and respect me within set boundaries.

Where the other staff members see me as one of them. And they do.

Really do, to the extent that I find myself telling my manager all about my mental health issues.

Why Holly, why?

He doesn't need to know.

All you've done is make a rod for your own back.

Worried that I'm letting my mental health define me, I decide to take action.

By giving my all. Inside and outside of therapy.

I aim to stop making myself sick.

But I can't stay at this weight.

I aim to stop self-harming.

But I need to let out my emotions.

I aim to open up more in appointments.

But I can't risk the rejection.

The evident rejection displayed by Graham constantly asking me if I've heard when the new treatment will start.

Obviously wants to get rid of me.

Probably for the best, as it's not like I talk much.

What is it that I always say?

New treatment, new start

So, I decide to give my all when I start at the personality disorder service.

I'm really starting to hate hope.

Seen as high functioning and because the waiting list is not getting shorter, I'm given the 'option' to join another group for treatment.

A weekly two-hour group therapy session run by two clinical psychologists and attended by up to 10 people with a range of difficulties including Obsessive Compulsive Disorder,

Personality Disorders, Post Traumatic Stress Disorder, Bipolar and Clinical Depression.

A lot less time and not condition or treatment specific as I want.

Talk about dangling a carrot in front of me then taking it away.

I'm told the choice is mine.

The stubborn part of me wants to wait for the personality disorder service. But its intensity means putting a halt to my life and that of my parents. It also means keeping Graham hanging on when we both know we are not going to get anywhere together.

I want to move on with my life.

I want to continue on the career trajectory.

I want to move out of my parents' house in the next year or two.

I want to be in an equal and stable relationship.

To do all of that I need to stop my pre conceptions of what it is I need, and just put my all into what comes my way.

So, I say yes to this two-year psychotherapy group.

But first, I need to be assessed for my suitability.

She doesn't seem to give two hoots about my history.

Only interested in what I want to gain from the group.

Isn't that obvious? Errr, to feel better perhaps.

She sets boundaries and expectations.

Including not to self-harm.

Right, okay.

If it were to come apparent that I was then I would be asked to leave the group immediately.

Woah hold your horses love. You think it's going to be that easy to stop. Just like that?

I leave the assessment with a potential start date in a few weeks' time, wondering what on earth I have let myself in for.

I may feel different. More mature if you like. Still, I can't shake of my feelings entering and my actions throughout the nutrition course at Plymouth eating disorder service. Worried that I'm going to do the same.

That nothing has changed.

CHAPTER 15

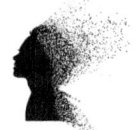

Entering the therapeutic room, I hang my head
in shame, remain silent and fiddle with what
is within my grasp.
With piercing eyes and an intuitive mind the
therapist silently opens my vulnerable soul
to the elements. Frozen to the chair for fear
of a slip of the tongue or an inappropriate
move cause's expression of physiological and
psychological tension. Disastrous images of
embarrassment flow rapidly in my mind being
excreted through blushing and sweating.
With the increasing volume of the imaginary
clock slowly ticking away, my head pounds
with every thought and feeling begging to be
released. Damaging my ability to dissociate,
I furiously scramble to gather these emotions
in a secure box before throwing away the key.

Acting according to protocol until I am a
good 100 yards away from the building saves

face and allows me to fractionise and store away the last hour. Not to be reminded of the session and my mental health difficulties, I goof off into "Holly world" where everything is pink and fluffy and recall does not exist. However, rumbling deep away in the depths of my mind and heart is the want and need to be emotionally expressive to confront my issues head on.

Hurting too much to accept, this desire gets caught up in my locked box of troubles.

Oh fuck.

The guy in the waiting room who attends a mental health resource centre I volunteered at, walks into the same therapy room as me.

Fuck.

He recognises me.

Double fuck.

With no choice, I act like I don't recognise him.

After all, I can't let him stop me from fully expressing myself and reaping any benefits this group may give me.

You're such a terrible person Holly: ignoring him in favour of your own needs.

Two girls in the group have had an eating disorder.

Don't let them beat you. Prove your worth. Lose weight.

One of who also has BPD. And self-harms as a result.

You got to be kidding me. I don't want to self-harm more.

But I do.

I cut just before each session. All the time thinking of the psychologist who told me that I can't do it.

With a smirk upon my face.

Afterwards feeling ashamed by the immaturity of my behaviour.

That I've completely let myself down yet again.

With my anger showing no signs of dissipating, I continue to act up.

I revel when the girl with BPD brings up the topic of suicide attempts and what would happen if we were to find ourselves in that situation.

Holly to the psychologists: 'So tell us, do we stop coming to these sessions? Will you give us extra support? Or will we just be dropped, as you know, that's not going to help us overcome our difficulties.'

Straight after another girl pipes up that she is trying to get extra support as this group is not enough for her.

The psychologists discomfort is obvious.

I bite my cheeks. Hard. Not that it wipes the smirk of my face.

Holly: 'Yea, I've been let down by all the services, especially during my last overdose, making the condemnation from my family so much harder to deal with.'

Why am I doing this?

Because they deserve it.

No, they don't. They are trying to help.

But they are not helping. You wouldn't be like this if they were. It's about time someone pays for all you've been through.

No. No one needs to pay for it. Blame is pointless. Focus on getting yourself better.

Before I have chance to think about my next steps, one of the psychologists addresses me directly. About my suicide attempt. Why I did it.

Why the fuck do you think? Stop accusing me of whatever it is you are.

Knowing his game, I stick to my well-rehearsed spiel.

He ain't getting nothing from me.

If it's a fight he wants, then it's a fight he'll get.

I've had enough of this group already.

It should be making me better. All it is doing is making me angrier.

I'm consumed with negative thoughts and am finding myself constantly acting out. Inside and outside of the group.

I need to curb this and quick smart.

Got our birthday coming up. AKA, got to be social.

Knowing that it was my mind trying to convince me of my family's desire to abandon me abroad less than six months ago, doesn't make Steven and mine upcoming holiday easier.

Nevertheless I throw myself into it, focusing on the positives.

So instead of thinking Steven' boyfriend insistence of driving us to the airport, crying when we leave, organising a surprise champagne bottle and chocolate bar in our hotel room (for Steven, not me) was his displeasure in us spending time together, I make myself think that it because he cares. Deeply. About Steven.

Rather than thinking Steven is trying to either starve me by not having breakfast, or fatten me up by insisting we eat dinner, I reason that he is wanting to keep us fuelled for our activities.

With renewed vigour, I look forward to continuing celebrating my birthday down Plymouth with friends.

Well, let's be honest, I'm more excited at the possibility of seeing Alan.

Seeing him will make me feel more secure. Not so out of place.

So as soon as I arrive, I text him.

I wait for a reply.

Nothing.

I text again.

Nothing.

I text once more.

Nothing.

I ask Noah if he knows where he is.

He has no idea.

I drink to blot out the pain.

I drink because he is not my only ex who isn't there.

Jasper no longer talks to me and Josh's new girlfriend has banned him from talking to, or seeing me.

I'm grateful for my friends being there. But I can't help feeling hurt that those who have been closet to me no longer want anything to do with me.

They must of seen something so dark and hideous in me that they can't bear to have me in their life anymore.

Perhaps my family deserve some credit for sticking by me then.

I give myself a pep talk.

People go their separate ways after University.

Maybe that's all this is.

Don't get caught up in feeling that you are losing people.

Do the same and move on with your life.

Focus on your career and people around you.

Of course, keep in touch with the friends you've made. Those who want you in their life will do the same.

This is natures course.

Go with it.

So I continue to go to therapy.

Not that it's much use.

I continue to go to work.

Not that I'm making much of a difference.

I continue to talk to and see friends.

Not convinced that they want to speak or spend time with me.

I continue to make effort with my family.

Still petrified that they could disown me at any given moment, without warning.

And for something new, I sign up to a dating website.

I find my inbox inundated with messages: the majority of which are cheesy and sexual.

Among them is a message from Albert.

We talk each day for an hour.

Living in London, we agree to meet up on my way back from seeing Gerty and Katie in the New Year.

Knowing I am going to see him gives me strength to cope with being away from home. From being somewhere where I have no control.

Somewhere where I'm confronted with people much skinner and much more jolly than me. Even if they are only ten years old.

Second day being down Somerset, Albert goes silent on me.

Instantly I know that something is up.

The day passes, as does the next day, without any contact with him.

My mind runs riot.

Why isn't he talking to me?

What is going on?

He hates me.

He doesn't want to meet up.

I've grossed him out.

Unable to escape these thoughts or the visual of that ten year old in my mind, sees me cut my arm. Over and over.

It's the day I go home. The day I meet Albert for the first time.

He texts.

Still wants to meet.

Relief washes over me and with that my mood stabilises.

Playing it cool I wait twenty minutes after arriving at Paddington station to text him.

An hour passes without a word from him.

I call.

Nothing.

Send a few more texts.

Nothing.

Two hours later I sullenly accept that he is not going to turn up. So I get up and make my way home. Silent tears falling down my face.

Needing to talk, but not to my family or friends, I open up in therapy.

Still worried about the potential ramifications if I were to say I've been self-harming, I make the decision not to mention it. That's until others disclose how hard they have found Christmas.

Why do I always have to 'one-up' others?

My admission is initially met with silence.

Oh fuck. Here we go. They are going to ask me to leave. Not that I care.

The psychologists ask why I did it and what I could do instead.

Holly: 'because I couldn't deal with my emotions. I don't know. Flick an elastic band on my wrist? Go for a walk? Write my thoughts and feelings down?'

The conversation then changes.

The session ends. They don't ask me to stay behind. So I wait for a phone call before the next session.

Nothing.

What does this mean? Am I still allowed to go back to the group?

Though unsure I'm welcome, I return to therapy, entering the room with trepidation.

As soon as we are all seated, the two psychologists talk.

They tell us that they need to talk to us about something.

That they understand self-harm is a symptom of some of our diagnosis's and that it can be hard to manage. However the point of therapy is to help us. To do that we need to help ourselves. So while the urge may be very real to us, it is important that we try not to engage in it. To find different ways to deal with the associated emotions.

I get it. I really do. But it's not easy: for us. And I guess, no, I know, it's not easy for them either.

So I agree. We all need to compromise. To meet half way. We, the service users, will try not to self-harm. The psychologists will be more understanding and try to better support us.

For years I have been bending myself backwards to please everyone and be what they want and need.

Recently, I've been uncompromising and inflexible. Demanding people to come to me. To sort me out. In effect, to be my savior.

Now, I see the need to meet in the middle. To give and take. For there to be balance.

Despite putting off meeting him for months, he still seems interested.

So I arrange to meet him.

Meet Evan from the dating website.

Force myself to go.

We meet in a pub round the corner from my house. You know, just in case.

He seems alright, albeit a bit too eager.

He wants to move on. To a different pub. I'm not too keen. But I've kept pushing him away. So I really should do something he wants.

He offers to drive.

Alarm bells ring in my head.

We are in his car.

The alarm bells are getting louder. Yet I ignore them.

We drive away from my home town. Out into the country.

No way I can get home on my own now. No money for a taxi either.

We walk into a pub. Order a drink.

He seems excited.

I have a drink to calm my nerves.

Still too early to call it a night, I order another. But drink slowly.

Ten o' clock comes and goes.

It's half ten. A decent time.

Holly: 'I really should be heading back. I've got work tomorrow.'

One more drink. Then we leave.

He drives me home.

I ask him to drive a bit further down from my house. I don't want my parents to see.

He takes it as I don't want my parents to see us kissing.

I don't want to kiss him. But he is staring at me.

Okay fine, a quick one.

He keeps at it. Keeps kissing me. Even when I don't give it my all.

Holly: 'I got to go.'

I don't leave immediately as I feel bad.

He takes that as a sign that I want to kiss him more. So he comes in for a kiss again.

Damn it Holly. You should of got up straight away.

I kiss him back.

I think to myself that it's nice to be wanted.

Holly: 'Right, I've got to go now.'

I turn to open the door, get up.

He says he will text me.

I know I don't want to see him again.

He is nice and all. Obviously happy and wants to be with me. But I'm just not into it.

Not wanting to hurt his feelings, I continue to talk to him: on and off. Not engaging in conversation that would indicate anything more than friendship.

At the same time I talk to other guys online.

One guy who is going through a tough time and just wants a friends with benefits relationship.

Another guy who simply wants no strings attached sex.

With none of the guys holding my interest, I decide to see who else has been looking at my profile.

A picture of a guy standing in between (who I presume to be) his grandparents, with his arms wrapped around them, pops up.

He is tall, rugby shaped with a big smile spread across his face.

I click on his profile. Look at his pictures. Read his blurb.

Then I see where he lives.

Great.

I leave it. But I can't stop thinking about him.

He mustn't be interested as he hasn't messaged him.

Shall I message him?

No, I can't. I am a girl. Men should make the first move.

He has. He has looked at your profile.

But he lives in Scotland, so it's pointless.

No harm in saying hi though.

So I do.

A few hours later he replies.

We get chatting.

He is currently living with his parents whilst writing up his PhD.

He has strong morals, close to his family, particularly his grandparents (the ones in the picture).

This is looking good.

Knowing that I'm setting myself up for disappointment but needing to know, I ask where he lives as I haven't heard of his town before.

Samuel: 'It's in Kent.'

In Kent? The county I live in? So not Scotland?

Straight away I go on google maps. Forty minutes' drive away.

Could this be it?

We continue to chat.

Frightened that I will spoil things, I let him lead. Let him suggest meeting up. Which he does, a few weeks later.

Of course the most suitable day is the day I have therapy.

Failing to skirt around that day, I decide to be honest.

Samuel: 'Shall I meet you outside afterwards?'

No trying to get out of it.

No questions about why I'm having therapy.

No silent treatment.

What is this?

Too good to be true is what it is.

I expect him not to turn up.

Ten minutes after our meeting time he calls. He is running a bit late due to traffic.

Crap, he is on his way.

Five more minutes pass. He drives up. In a mini. The old mini. A proper nice, well looked after old mini.

That's a well nice car, but he mustn't be as tall as his picture made him out to be.

He gets out of the car.

My mistake.

He greets me, opens the passenger door. I get in, see a bunch of flowers on the back seat.

There's no chance in hell a guy like this will ever like me. But what an experience this will be.

We end up in the local Weatherspoon's.

Talk for three hours straight.

Discuss what we want. Relationship? Marriage? Kids? Career?

We are on the same page.

He is so darn beautiful.

His eyes and smile enchant me.

He is the right height and width to hold me in his arms. Tightly and safely.

He speaks the Queen's English.

He is smart, strong and stable.

He is just… well, no words.

Don't think too much into it.

Don't get carried away.

Leave the ball in his court.

It pays off.

We go on a second date to a national trust site.

I pay for parking as he drove.

Equality. I like it.

I accidentally fling mud at him. He doesn't seem put off.

We arrange a third date where he asks me to go to his friend's wedding reception with him.

Oh G*d. What am I going to wear? What are they going to think of me? Will I meet everyone's standard?

Parked outside my parents later that night he tells me he thinks he is starting to fall in love with me.

I go silent.

No one has said this to me before.

Samuel:' You don't need to say it back.'

Holly: 'I think I feel the same.'

Taking the bullet by the horn, I ask if we are official.

Samuel: 'Yes.'

Wow. I can't breathe.

We kiss.

Getting harder to breathe.

———

Things seem to be changing. Quickly and for the better.

But a big part of me still feels numb. In fact, empty.

Refusing to let this ruin things, I push forwards, focusing on what I can do and what will benefit myself and others.

First of all, I set up an education and career group as well as develop a newsletter with the residents at work.

Secondly, I continue working on my relationships with family, friends and Samuel.

Thirdly, I widen my net in the job market.

I go for an assistant psychologist interview at a private healthcare firm.

They offer me the job.

This is everything you wanted. Take it. Take it now.

Wait a minute.

Am I ready?

Ready to move out of home?

Ready to move away from a relationship. The first adult relationship I've had?

Ready to leave therapy?

Ready to have this level of responsibility?

Unsure, I seek out advice. For the first time.

Wow, change really is happening.

I ask Mum, Steven, Samuel, Gemma and Gerty what they think.

Ultimately the decision lies with me.

Ultimately I know what I got to do.

I turn it down.

Undeterred, I continue to apply for other jobs. Both local and national.

I go to an interview for a trainee Psychological Wellbeing Practitioner (PWP) post.

I make it to first reserve.

News that the company I work for is being re-structured makes me want this job even more.

My manager offers me a senior role in another service. But it's in a different county.

I could either move or commute.

I don't want to do either.

Mainly because of the potential impact it may have on my relationship with Samuel. But also because I just don't want it.

Mum: 'You should take it. You've made huge leaps in treatment over the last year and it would be a shame to miss out on the offer from a manager who strongly believes in you.'

Yea, okay. But I don't want it.

Not wanting to shoot myself in the foot, I tell them I will think about it. That I will give them an answer when I get back from holiday.

A holiday I don't want to, nor have the money to go on.

But I do.

I do because its Gerty's first holiday abroad with friends.

I do, because Gerty will need someone to help her. That person is me.

So I try to force myself to enjoy the tightly scheduled activities. Activities that I would not chose to do on my holidays.

Needing a break, I tell Gerty and Katie that I'm going to give the zoo a miss.

What a grave mistake that is.

Katie lays into me.

With no energy I relent. No, I more than relent. I make a joke of it. I say I am over-tired but if they want me to go then I will.

Katie: 'Yes, you need to come.'

Fine, whatever.

Katie also insists that I go swimming with them.

No chance in hell.

Taking a lot, I tell them that I don't feel comfortable wearing a swimming costume.

Katie: 'Nor do I, but I am going to go swimming because Gerty wants to.'

Woah! Firstly, Gerty can speak for herself. She says it is fine if I don't want to go swimming.

Secondly, this is about me and not you.

Thirdly, this is as much my holiday as it is both of yours.

Fourthly, you have no right demanding anything of me, especially because you know how I feel about myself.

Why does Katie think she can tell me what to do and that I will do what she says?

Though thankful for being back home, I know I need to start facing my demons. Not waiting for someone to face them for me.

First step is to ask for help and this time mean it.

So I take Samuel up on his offer.

His offer to ask me to stop self-harming.

Samuel: 'Will you stop self-harming.'

Holly: 'Okay.'

I also ask him for help with my eating when I'm with him. To eat healthily and the right amount of food.

I'm not quite ready for him to ask me not to make myself sick.

I can't give everything to him in one go. I need some form of control.

The assumption that this means we will have a perfect relationship is soon shown for what it is.

A delusion.

Because I will always do something to ruin it.

First of all I pull out of going to see Coldplay with him at the last minute due to extreme anxiety at not knowing how to act when I'm there.

Do I stand? Sit? Jump up and down? G*d forbid, sing?

What will Samuel expect of me?

Second of all, I embarrass Samuel at another one of his friend's wedding.

Firstly, by wearing an outfit that I spend weeks looking for. An outfit which he says I look nice in, but one where he gives off vibes of not liking it.

Secondly, not clicking with his girl friends who I'll be sitting with during the ceremony. Evident in being left standing on my own whilst they go off with one another.

Thirdly, being forced to get up on the dance floor. Not

knowing what to do and full of shame and embarrassment, I just stand there.

Third of all, I screw up meeting him before we go watch the Olympic canoe slalom in Lee Valley.

I wait for him at his local station for half an hour with a dead phone. I ask the staff if they have a phone charger.

They do.

I plug my phone in and turn it on.

Missed calls and messages from Samuel fill my screen.

He is at his waiting for me. Apparently where we agreed to meet.

I call.

He is annoyed but comes to pick me up.

We still have time to get to the Olympics.

Whilst I wait, I pick up a voicemail.

I've been offered the trainee PWP job.

The job that combines studying for a post-graduate certificate whilst undertaking clinical practice. Meaning that I get the best of both worlds: further academic training and hands on clinical experience.

Without thinking twice I take it.

Mainly because Samuel works in the same county twice a week.

Also because it means I don't need to take the job my manager has offered.

I tell Samuel when he picks me up.

Though still annoyed, he is happy for me.

Is this our first argument?

I say goodbye to the staff and residents at work.

Feeling gratitude to them all.

Having only completed six months of the two year programme, I say goodbye to everyone in therapy, and to therapy itself.

Content that it is the right time and the right thing to do.

I say goodbye to my parents and my family home. Knowing that now I'm moving out for good, I will not be allowed to move back in.

Feeling strong and ready to stand on my own two feet.

I say goodbye to Samuel, knowing that I will see him two days a week when he comes up to work.

Not knowing for sure what will happen in our relationship, but settling for being okay no matter the outcome.

CHAPTER 16

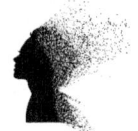

I'M ON MY OWN. Feeling separated from everyone.

I'm forced to make the effort. With others and with myself.

I put myself forward with my new colleagues whilst still keeping in touch with old friends and family.

I refer myself to the University disability service just in case I need extra support.

I join the gym.

I spend my evenings either doing homework or reading.

I see Samuel regularly. Soon enough I see him every day as he moves in after getting a one year fixed term job near me.

Moves in after making the comment that if we can't live together then it would be an end to the relationship.

Makes total sense.

So what do I have to do?

Act as the perfect girlfriend.

What does this entail?

Be what he wants me to be.

Pre-empt his every thought, wish and desire to make sure he is happy all the time.

Do absolutely everything and anything as not to cause a disagreement, or heaven forbid, an argument.

Not to have my own opinion unless I'm sure it is one he agrees with.

Do as he asks.

We go to see one of Samuels friends who lives nearby. A friend he has told about my mental health issues.

Which I am fine with. After all he did ask me before he told her.

He tells me that she wants to meet me and know more about me, particularly my mental health. But only if I want to talk about it.

I'm not sure I do.

But it's the first time I will be meeting her. She's a good friend of Samuel's. Maybe it will help me?

So I tell her. She's interested. Really interested.

I don't feel judged. But I also don't feel relieved.

I just hope that I'm not going to be seen as Samuel's girl-friend who has mental health issues.

Now living together and expected as well as wanting to contribute equally, I feel that I'm left with no choice but to take Samuel up on his previous suggestion.

To get myself a debt management plan.

This means pushing past the stereotypes that I have of those in debt as well as the embarrassment of asking for his help and having to reveal the extent of my debt to him.

With the plan set up I also have to contend with the embar-rassment of not being able to afford any spontaneous social activities, or any activities that cost more than a tenner at a time.

So no more birthday holidays with Steven.

No takeaways.

No celebrations.

I'm destined to live a life of desolation.

Or so I think.

Samuel offers to lend me money so I can go to one of my sisters hen dos, and for Steven and mine birthday meal with Mum and Dad.

He tells me he doesn't expect me to pay him back straight away.

It's a nice act. I know it is. But I can't help thinking that this is him trying to control me. Control what events I can and can't go to. Controlling me by me being in his debt.

So not only do I need to be the perfect girlfriend, I got to be a dependent one.

I fall easily into the role of a dependent girlfriend.

Despite knowing that it is not what I want.

Also despite knowing that it is not what Samuel wants.

But knowing that it is the easiest and safest road for me.

Because with it comes a lack of responsibility. A lack of responsibility in making decisions. Where you simply do what you are told without argument.

So coming home after work to find Samuel making paper chains for Christmas sees me dutifully join in rather than express upset that he has done this without me.

Doesn't matter that he is doing it as a surprise.

Feeling guilty that Samuel is only invited to the evening party at my sister's wedding means that I have no choice but to wait to fully enjoy myself until he arrives.

Can't let him think that I can have a good time without him.

Not understanding that I need a bit of time to myself whilst staying at his parents for a few days over Christmas, sees Samuel tell me 'that I should go home' if I'm not going to be social.

My silent cries sees him apologies, yet I can't stand up for myself and tell him how he has made me feel and why I need time on my own.

Unable to afford it, I cancel my plans to see Gemma in the New Year. Samuel also cancels his plans to see his friends. So we stay at home, watching Jools Holland and drinking champagne.

Fear of him thinking how different we are means that I can't tell him that I don't enjoy these two things.

THE MONSTER in my head is metamorphosing from myself to Samuel. Where I battle against him and not myself.

He is the one who is bringing trouble and destruction.

And he does.

Well, he does until he doesn't.

When he picks me up and stops me wallowing in self-pity.

A month after sitting my role play exam, it is confirmed that I have failed it.

Failed because I had forgotten to ask one question.

Doesn't matter that I'm not the only one.

Also doesn't matter that I have the chance to re-sit.

This fail dictates my ability as a practitioner and defines my character. Both of which are negative.

Not taking it, Samuel forces me out of bed, to shower, to go to town and treats me to a hot chocolate.

It works.

He is not the monster that my mind is making him out to be.

With renewed confidence, I spend my spare time revising and practicing the role play with course mates.

I resit the exam, leaving thirty minutes later sure that I have done enough to pass.

Yea right.

It takes a whole month to find out that I have failed once again.

Fuck.

This can't be happening.

All my life I've wanted to be a therapist.

Now it looks like I am not good enough to be one.

My life is over. Like seriously over.

I stop eating.

I'm told to apply for extenuating circumstances.

Despite not using the disability service much, I'm told to ask them to support my case.

For some reason unbeknown to me, they do.

Now I have to wait.

Thirty-one hours have passed without eating.

I'm at a quiz with Samuel and his friends.

I'm expected to eat.

Being dutiful, I do.

I do, but enforce Plan B.

Plan B being taking myself to the toilet straight after and making myself sick. With my fingers as I don't have my toothbrush on me.

My phone rings the next morning.

It's my supervisor. She's heard that I failed. She tells me to take the next two days off.

Fuck. I'm going to lose my job.

Unable to cope, I stay in bed all morning.

In the afternoon I go to the shop and buy chocolate, crisps and ice cream.

I stuff it all in my mouth.

Before my body has chance to digest it all, I make myself sick.

Not enough, and feeling empty, I raid the cupboards and gorge on the breakfast bars.

I make myself sick again.

Of course Samuel wants one when he gets home.

I burst into tears having broken my previous promise to him that I wouldn't binge on them.

Not a dutiful girlfriend after all.

I tell him that I've been either starving or binging followed by making myself sick.

He takes me in his arms.

Where's this monster?

He suggests not having any of the bars in the house.

There it is!

He suggests having smaller and healthier portions at meal times.

He thinks I'm fat!

He tells me he will do the same.

No, you won't. you're a man, you have to eat more than me.

This monster has evolved.

It plays with me. One minute being nice. The next being horrible.

I know the monster isn't Samuel.

But it's easier to give it a form. A form that isn't me.

And it's much easier when Samuel does things I don't like but don't have the power to speak up about.

⸺

IT'S the day that Katie and Gerty come up for the weekend.

Arriving early, Samuel makes me go and meet Katie rather than wait until Gerty arrives.

We go for a drink.

Katie berates me at not telling her something I knew before her.

She also berates me for not visiting her.

Surprisingly I stand my ground. I tell her that I do not break what I am told in confidence and I explain the extent of my financial strain.

It does the trick.

Maybe I can tell people what I think.

Maybe I should speak freely to Samuel. That way I won't see him as a monster.

It's not just Katie out to get me. It's Gerty's Mum as well.

She tells me she has paid for Katie and I to have breakfast for the two days they are here.

With no choice but to comply, my hand is forced yet again to make myself sick afterwards.

I spend the rest of the weekend praying for it to be over.

Thankfully it comes quick.

Desperate to meet Samuel, I drop Katie of at the station knowing that she doesn't want to go home.

As soon as I meet Samuel, Katie texts saying she has missed her train.

He forces me to go and get her. Bring her to the pub until the next train.

I really need a break.

She bursts into tears.

In front of Samuel she says how I haven't been supporting her. How I am living the life of Riley all because I have completed University, no longer live with my parents and have a boyfriend.

This is all Samuel's fault. He shouldn't of told me to go get her, especially because I know that she has missed her train on purpose.

I reiterate my situation to Katie.

My debt.

Still suffering with mental health.

At risk of failing my course.

Some of my relationships still being strained.

This seems to placid Katie. More so when Samuel confirms the situation.

Feeling better now she knows my life isn't perfect, Katie gets the train home.

CHAPTER 17

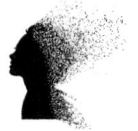

As the hours tick by my stomach growls louder
and my mind grows weaker.

Overcoming the hurdles of the first few days
will bring the joy that I desperately
desire. Pro-Ana websites and pictures of
thin stars are used as reinforcers. Feelings
of nausea and weakness suddenly wash over me,
convincing me of the need to eat. I stuff my
face with nutritionally bad items before my
mind has a chance to fight back. Feeling
full, I stop and asses what I have done.
Toothbrush in tow, I head to the bathroom,
expelling the evil that I have let inside
of me.

Feeling drained, I curl up in bed lost and
alone. Silent tears stream down my face
filled with memories of time gone by.
Summers spent running around the garden with

my siblings, playing cat's cradle with my Mum
and drawing trains with my Dad.   I'm
pampered with the smell of roses, the sight
of trees blooming and the sound of birds
singing their song.
Not a cloud in the sky, not a care in the
world.

The memory vanishes as the tear falls from my
chin. I'm flung back into the present, to the
sorrow that gladly surrounds me. Starring at
the four walls containing me, a sigh of utter
loss rises from deep inside. For a fraction
of a second, part of the pain is lessened.
I stare motionless at the remnants lingering
in the air, my body without sensation.
A sharp tug of air brings me back into a
reality I would rather not face.

⊏⊐

My career is still hanging by a thread.

My relationships feel unstable.

My mind continues to make Samuel out to be a monster, despite contradictory evidence.

I have no idea what is going on and I definitely have no control over it.

So the cycle of starvation, binging and vomiting continues.

The self-harming would be there to, if it wasn't for promising Samuel that I'd stop.

Just keep swimming.

Just keep swimming.

Just keep swimming swimming swimming.

What do we do we swim swim swim.

So that's what I do.

I make myself accept the situation.

The situation of having my clients taken off me and having to shadow my colleagues whilst I wait for the outcome of my second and final resit.

I make myself attend events when all I'd rather do is stay in bed.

I make myself feign enjoyment and happiness at things I should even though I feel anything but that.

So I go to my Nan's seventieth birthday meal. I eat and mingle with family, pretending that everything is okay.

I sit the Lancaster University clinical psychology doctorate exam knowing that I won't do well enough to get offered an interview. Which I don't.

Samuel and I celebrate our one year anniversary. He surprises me with a trip to London and an overnight stay at a posh hotel in Green Park. Whilst I still can't believe my luck at being with him, I can't help but feel empty.

I resit the role play exam. And pass.

I go to my cousins wedding despite feeling awkward as we haven't spoken much since we hit our teenage years.

I go to the Cardiff University interview for the clinical doctorate. I'm not offered a place.

That's fine. I'm not ready for it. Plus it would mean moving away from Samuel. In fact it would mean ending our relationship as prior experience has shown him that long distance relationships don't work.

Obviously I'm not worth trying it again for.

With training almost over and knowing that I don't want to stay working for this service, I apply for qualified PWP jobs.

I get offered numerous interviews, but take up the first job offer.

It's a two hour commute each way, but it means I can stay with Samuel. More than that, it is a place I get good vibes from, and it's a place where I can start afresh.

And I do start afresh.

Having all but gotten away without needing any extra support for my mental health issues in the last year shows me that I am better.

A lack of money due to the debt management plan and with Samuel keeping an eye on me, means that I no longer have the means to binge. And as I can't do that, the likelihood that I will make myself sick afterwards reduces.

I do not have the willpower, strength or energy to starve myself for long periods of time anymore.

As a qualified practitioner I am closer to achieving my dreams of being a clinical psychologist, therefore feel that I have not wasted the last nine years of my life.

I haven't taken an overdose in over a year nor cut in just under a year.

More determined than ever not to let my mental health define me, I decide not to tell anyone at work. Not occupational health and not my colleagues.

Though risky, they can make their judgements about me based on my performance and personality.

I've got this.

To maintain being strangely okay at a size fourteen, I force myself to the gym two to three times a week and to eat healthily. Though trying not to be angry at Samuel for making me eat tones of vegetables and salad takes some doing on the days I just want to feel free from the eating disorder. To eat what I want without feeling bad for it. To have the money to be able to do that.

Niggling voice: 'If you weren't with him, you could eat what you want, when you want. Spend money as and how you see fit. In essence, you wouldn't need to follow his commands or report back to him.

'No. this is not what he is doing. He is helping me. Introducing me to new and healthy foods to combat my issues with food. He is showing me how to eat and maintain a healthy body weight. Something I have never been able to do, and something nobody else has been able to help me do.

Niggling voice: 'if that's what you think. Time will tell.'

⊏══⊐

The battle in my head is exhausting. Particularly when it tries to pin the blame on Samuel. Nevertheless I continue to fight on.

I fight it by putting work before it.

By putting relationships before it.

More importantly, by putting my unknown future before it.

All of which seem to work.

I'm getting on well with all my colleagues. They appear to like me.

I am developing well in my job, narrowly winning the competition to recruit the highest number of patients to a digital mental health and wellbeing service.

I'm offered two interviews for the doctorate in clinical psychology and am invited to apply for a PhD with the program director of the Masters I took.

I go to one of the doctorate interviews and the PhD interview.

I'm offered the latter the same day.

I consider whether to take it and whether to go to the other doctorate interview.

Samuel: 'If you get a place there, it would put a strain on our relationship but we could try.'

At least he is not saying it would mean an end to our relationship.

Samuel: 'We can look to moving half way between Berkshire and Bournemouth if you take the PhD.'

Well, it's a no brainer. I'm taking the PhD.

Not even going to go to the other interview.

Samuel first.

Despite my heart lying in clinical work.

Despite what feels like insurmountable fears in my ability to conduct research.

Think of the silver lining Holly.

Your heart may be in clinical, but given your own struggles, it may not be the right path for you. Not yet.

Remember that being offered a PhD with a studentship is an achievement in itself.

You can always apply for the clinical doctorate after the PhD, when hopefully you are in a more stable place.

With the decision made, we start looking for a place to live.

We move six weeks before my PhD starts.

Still working in London, I stay with Steven in the weekdays and spend weekends visiting friends, family and Samuel.

———

Living at Steven's, I do not have access to a gym.

Knowing the importance of exercise on my wellbeing, I start doing home workouts daily.

Sit ups, push-ups, jumping jacks and stretches to name a few.

Aware of my decrease in exercise and not having money to pay Steven rent or to buy my own food, means that I only eat at dinner time.

I also stop eating junk food.

Cakes, crisps, chocolate, ice cream, fizzy drinks, sweets, biscuits, chips.

Nothing deters me from this path. Not even going on holiday to celebrate Julie and Laura's thirtieth birthday.

A cheap holiday I can afford from a tax rebate.

I worry that time apart from Samuel will make him fall out of love with me. Or will make him realise that he never loved me in the first place.

So getting off the train at Winchester feels me with trepidation.

I walk along the station platform and see Samuel waiting for me.

Tears spring to my eyes.

My heart suddenly and painfully aches for him.

I get closer to him.

I see him smiling at me.

I throw my arms around him.

Holly: 'I've missed you.'

I'm verbally expressing my emotions now?

Samuel: 'I've missed you too.'

It suddenly hits me.

This is what love feels like.

We go home. First time I've been there since we signed contracts.

Our furniture is there. Both old and the new ones we have ordered.

It's homely. He has made it homely. For us.

He loves me.

Lighting can strike twice.

———

We are paying more rent.

Our bills are more expensive.

I'm taking an £8,000 pay cut.

I've got another three years on the debt management plan.

So it helps that Samuel has been given a permanent contract where he works.

But it means that I really can't afford anything.

Not even to join the gym.

I tell Samuel that it's fine. That I can continue my home workouts.

It doesn't wash with him, but it's what needs to happen.

So, I push it to the back of my mind and focus on starting my PhD journey with a bang.

Samuel meets me in town after the first day.

Unable to stop it, I burst into tears.

He doesn't get it.

He loved his first day of his PhD. He loved all of his PhD journey.

I bet he wasn't made to feel like an outcast.

I bet he wasn't told to work in a different office by a fellow student as there was not enough space in the office he was meant to be in.

Don't let this get you down Holly. Fight it.

So I speak to the technician.

He finds a desk for me.

I move in.

Start to get to know the other students.

The girls are bitchy and the boys keep themselves to themselves.

Didn't realise I was back in the playground.

Weeks pass and I still don't know what I am doing with the PhD.

I'm struggling to connect with my peers.

Though doing home workouts daily, I find it hard not being able to go to the gym.

Both Samuel and I are worn out from our long commutes.

Something needs to give.

Food.

I tell myself that it's okay to have a packet of crisps.

I tell myself they only cost 60p a packet.

I tell myself that I can afford it as I get to keep the money from marking undergraduate essays.

I tell myself that the crisps are only 179 calories.

I tell myself that that's okay as I haven't had breakfast.

I tell myself that I don't need to eat lunch if I have them.

I tell myself that I will be eating healthy dinners with Samuel.

I tell myself that my daily workouts amount to more calorie loss than the crisps hold.

I tell myself that as no one can see you eat them you have to have them as soon as you get to the office.

I convince myself that this is okay.

Soon enough I convince myself that two packets of crisps are okay.

Two packets of crisps and a chocolate bar.

I start to feel guilty for eating them.

I start to feel self-disgust.

I start to feel I'm letting Samuel down.

I start to get angry at people.

Particularly those who randomly turn up in the office before me, or whilst I'm scoffing my face.

Particularly at Samuel for telling me I can't join the gym and for leaving me with no money.

I know that I am not putting on weight, therefore do not need to stop what I am doing or to make myself sick.

I know that I am not harming anyone as nobody knows what I am doing or commenting on the effect it is having on them or me.

Samuel: 'If you really want to go to the gym, then maybe you can sign up in the New Year. Use the money you get from marking.'

I know Samuel is not saying this because he is aware of what I am doing.

He is saying it because he hates me. Thinks I'm disgusting and that I am not good enough for him.

My colossal need to go back to the gym ever so slightly outweighs my anger at Samuel.

Holly: 'Yea sure, that's a good idea.'

Why is he telling me what to do with my money?

Why do I need his permission?

He does not own me or control me. I am joining the gym because I want to. Not because he says so.

So on the first January 2015, I join the gym.

They offer an induction and three free personal training sessions.

I take it up. Refuse to be weighed but agree for them to measure my waist, arms and legs as a guide in my weight loss journey.

I'm shocked at the width of my waist.

I'm fat. I'm actually fat.

Vowing to change this, I force myself to the gym four days a week.

I continue with my home workouts seven days a week. Adding, different plank variations, squats and lunges to my routine.

A routine that takes thirty minutes to complete.

I get up with Samuel at five in the morning.

Do my home workout as soon as he leaves for work.

Going to the gym straight after if it's his non-gym day.

On his gym days, I wait to go with him when he gets back from work. Stressed and anxious just in case he changes his mind. Leaving me to go to the gym on my own at the busiest time.

Where people will stare at me.

⌷

I start a healthy eating routine.

Breakfast: Porridge with raisins or Weetabix with cinnamon and a banana.

Lunch: Homemade salad consisting of lettuce leaf's, spinach, sweetcorn, pepper, carrots, radish, tomatoes, beetroot, cucumber, croutons with salad dressing and a mix of seeds and nuts. An apple and/or banana after.

Dinner: Vegetarian meal high in protein, low in carbohydrates with plenty of vegetables.

My one woman mission where failure doesn't exist is taking form.

I'm losing centimetres from my waist, arms and legs.

My clothes are getting bigger on me.

I start to fit into small size twelve jeans.

I'm getting fitter.

I'm also getting on with some of my peers and not caring about those who I do not gel with.

My research is taking direction. The direction I want it to take.

I present my work at the department conference, winning first place in the oral presentation.

I'm getting papers published.

More than this, and much more important than this is the fact that I am throwing my weight loss in Laura's face.

Laura, who I told to get me a size fourteen bridesmaid dress for her wedding in nine months' time, has gone and bought me a size eighteen online.

I have never been a size eighteen. Well, I was bordering on a size eighteen nine years ago.

A whole nine years ago.

Honestly what is she thinking?

Wanting to hurt me is what is going through her mind.

Nevertheless, my healthy routine makes me start to feel gratitude.

Gratitude towards Samuel.

For helping me eat healthily.

For suggesting I use my marking money to join the gym.

I feel closer to me.

We are closer.

So close that we talk about our future.

We not only talk about buying our own place, we actively look into it.

Start saving for a deposit.

Attend 'Help to Buy' events.

Talk about getting married after we've bought a home.

Of course this happiness doesn't last for long.

CHAPTER 18

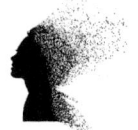

Not allowing me to move past a year of a
healthy mind and body, you decide to
indirectly attack me.
Using my biggest weakness to your advantage
wasn't enough for you. You pushed me to blame
myself for the pain of someone close
experiencing exactly what I've been through.
Being two peas in a pod, it wasn't just the
behaviours and negative thoughts that were
striking in similarity. Our deepest fears and
concerns that opens the spiral were mirrored.
Convincing me that the only way to help was
to self-punish, I was left with no choice.
Thoughts of slicing my throat and stomach
open came flooding back. Starving to binging,
to making myself sick became a daily
occurrence. Upping my exercise regime and
pushing myself harder in work led to failure
paving the way for me to end it all.

My increased emotional resilience wasn't enough for me to fight you. My tortured soul returned with a vengeance. No longer able to brush aside or ignore the strong emotional responses intensified the mental and physical ramifications of your presence. Being relentless in pushing me harder every day led to physical damage to my body coming thick and fast.

Unable to stop yet scared of damaging myself further, I'm left hating myself for having to self-punish as a result of being a despicable human being.

I have a feeling that she is going through a hard time.

But I just don't want to know.

I can't know.

So I shut myself off from it as long as is possible.

But as soon as she tells me, that is it.

Handling the situation the only way I know how, sees me be there for her by hurting myself.

A big part of me hates her for it.

But a bigger part of me wants to save her.

Whether it will or not is not the point. It's something I need to do. Something I have no choice in.

So I start to skip breakfast

Stop eating fruit after my salad.

Not finish all my dinner. Telling Samuel that I am full.

I push myself harder at the gym. Sometimes I go twice a day.

And I start making myself sick again.

I cut down on hot chocolates.

Knowing this, Samuel takes me to a juice bar instead.

I battle with myself on the way there and when ordering.

I tell myself that I need to drink it despite not wanting to.

Samuel: 'You've been really quiet recently. What's going on?'

Holly: 'Nothing.'

We sit in silence.

I try to smile at Samuel.

He's not fooled.

Tears form in my eyes.

Tell him Holly.

Whispering I tell him I've started to make myself sick again.

I hang my head low.

I take a risk and glance up at him.

He doesn't look surprised.

I tell him about Gemma and how it has made me relapse.

I tell him that I am controlling what I eat more.

That I want to self-harm, but am resisting.

Then before I know it, three words come out of my mouth.

Holly: 'I need help.'

Samuel asks me to make a promise to him.

Holly: 'I promise to try not to make myself sick.'

I also promise to only go to the gym three times a week and to eat three meals a day.

I do as is asked and as I promise.

Feeling more and more despondent as the days go by.

In a further bid to help, Samuel invites Gemma down without me knowing.

He takes her number from my phone and organise it.

I panic.

I can't have her down here. She can't see me like this. She can't be here given what she is going through.

Why the hell has he invited her down?

Well, it's not like she will come, as I'm the one who has always gone to hers, rather than her come to me.

But she does

She seems well.

She makes me laugh.

Says she is happy to see me eating.

And I am happy to see her.

Why am I happy to see her? I should be mad that she is here.

Mad because with her here I feel that it is okay to eat. And I can't feel like that because I got Laura's wedding to go to.

I continue to eat when Gemma has gone.

I continue to eat in spite of panicking that I'm going to end up in that size eighteen bridesmaid dress.

Not because that is the dress I got, but because that is the dress size that fits me.

I continue to eat despite Mum paying and ordering the same dress in a size twelve for me.

Yup, smaller than I initially thought!

And I continue to eat up to and on the day of Laura's wedding.

I eat fearing that the fuss I made about the dress needing to be a size fourteen begin thrown in my face when it doesn't fit.

But I can't stop eating. Despite the immense terror it brings with it.

I can't stop because I'm stuck in a routine.

Routine of three healthy meals a day, gym three to four times a week and home workouts seven days a week.

Also the routine of studying for my PhD, paying off my debt, being with Samuel and applying for shared ownership properties.

A routine that also involves celebrating events.

This time Steven and mine thirtieth Birthday.

We decide to go to Centre Parcs with our partners.

A place where I can continue my routine of healthy eating and exercise.

Julie also comes. Laura says she can't afford it.

I know I am in a good routine. A healthy routine.

It's a routine that is seeing things change for the better.

But I'm not coping.

How?

How can I still not be coping?

Despite moving back to Berkshire in a few months, I decide to take the bull by the horn.

I go and see my GP.

She agrees I need psychological support but tells me its best to get it when I move.

She offers anti-depressants in the meantime.

No thanks. Didn't work last time. Won't work this time.

So I wait.

In the meantime I prepare for my transfer exam for my PhD and my talk at the Eating Disorder Awareness week at the University.

I'm surprisingly confident before the transfer.

I'm surprisingly confident during the transfer.

I'm somewhat dumbstruck with the outcome.

They tell me there's disparity in what I've written and what I've said.

They ask me to re submit

Oh shit. My gut instinct before I took the PhD was right. I can't do this.

Examiner: 'Could you be dyslexic?'

Excuse me?

Do I look like I have a learning disability?

Apparently so.

She suggests I go and get assessed.

Dutiful as ever, I go as soon as they release me.

With no time to dwell, I prepare for my talk on eating disorders.

I feel okay about it.

Okay with my ability to talk about my experiences.

That's until I get there and find myself waiting outside with the audience.

The audience who keeps coming.

I start to shake.

My breathing becomes shallow.

Deep breathes Holly. In and out. In and out.

I give myself a pep talk as I walk into the room and set up.

You gave a talk about eating disorders just last week to the local radio station.

You have spoken to MSc students about eating disorders.

You've got this. You know you have.

Ready to go, I look up at the audience.

Oh fuck. There's a lot of them.

I take a deep breathe, re-focus and start.

Holly: 'Hi, my name is Holly. Today I will be talking about emotions as the backbone to eating disorders.'

Before I know it, it's over.

I've given my talk, answered questions and had my photo taken.

I return back to Winchester . My last night there before joining Samuel in our own home.

Goodbye Winchester

Hello Bracknell.

Starting as I mean to go on, I book an induction at the gym and see my new GP.

She refers me to the common point of entry team for assessment.

They ask if I want to be referred to the eating disorder service or the personality disorder service.

I opt for the former.

I go and see them, leaving with a new diagnosis. This time Eating Disorder Not Otherwise Specified (EDNOS).

I also go for an assessment with an educational psychologist.

He confirms that I have both dyslexia and dyspraxia.

Both are mild forms, but still.

Bloody genes.

What next? Are they going to tell me I'm also autistic?

Might as well diagnosis me with everything else whilst they are at it.

Though I'm pissed off that there is something else wrong with me and that it has taken thirty years to be picked up on, I tell myself not to look a gift horse in the mouth. After all they are offering support in the form of assistive technology and for me to work with a tutor assessor and a specialist mental health mentor.

Support that helps me pass my transfer. Meaning that I am one step closer in getting a PhD.

⊏▭⊐

I feel pressure.

Pressure of waiting to start treatment at the eating disorder service.

And with that pressure of being unwell enough to qualify for treatment.

Pressure of being a bridesmaid at Julie's wedding.

Particularly as I can't escape my head telling me that I caused nothing but issues in the run up to Laura's wedding.

Pressure at making friends where I live.

And with that, fear of being isolated.

Especially because I study in a different county, work from home a lot and failed to make friends while living in Winchester, so will likely fail here.

So, to be accepted for treatment, not cause Julie problems and to make friends, I join the local netball team and start going to yoga.

I also hire a personal trainer having spare money since finishing paying off my debt.

The netball girls and the personal trainer are nice. But I don't form a connection with any of them.

I'm still alone.

Must try harder.

So I push myself when exercising but end up with a knee injury.

I ask the personal trainer for a food plan.

I remind him that I want to lose weight and about my history with eating disorders.

My trust in him is misplaced.

My clothes are getting tighter.

I'm turning into the hulk.

I exercise more to counteract the rising anxiety and panic in me.

My knee injury gets worse.

I get fatter.

I see a physiotherapist who advices me to stop playing netball for a while.

I don't.

I struggle to bend my knee and walk without a limp.

She tells me to stop again.

I do.

There's obviously no point in trying to improve myself when all it does is make things worse.

Makes things worse in terms of me getting fatter and becoming more socially inept.

———

Whether he knew I was getting worse…

Whether he simply wanted a holiday…

Or whether he wanted us to go away together again like we used to…

Steven offers to pay for a mini holiday away for us. Just the two of us.

He shouldn't pay for me.

I'm thirty-one. I'm an adult. I'm self-sufficient.

But I don't have spare money.

I want to spend time with him. I miss him. I miss our holidays together.

I tell myself that the only way I can go and be just a little bit okay with him paying for it, is if I open up to him whilst there.

Oh G*d, oh G*d, oh G*d.

So I tell him.

I tell him about my recent efforts to meet new people, to exercise properly via a personal trainer. Hoping it will kick my eating disorder in the butt. But also hoping that it won't. That it will make me worse.

Make me worse by making me skinner. Which will also make me better.

I tell him how my personal training sessions make me feel.

Steven: 'it might just be your body shape changing.'

Holly: 'Yes, but it's making me put on weight. My clothes are not fitting like thy used to. It's making my issues worse.'

Steven: 'Maybe you need to stop the food plan and not see the trainer anymore. What you were doing before was working.'

With his approval, I put an end to it.

I stop the food plan. Going back to eating the three healthy meals a day.

I tell my personal trainer that I am stopping our sessions. Using my studying as an excuse as not to hurt his feelings.

But I take his two High Intensity Training (HIT) workouts and incorporate them into my home workout routines.

I also carry on with some of the strength and resistance training exercises he taught me, but mix it with more cardio.

On a role, I decide to stop netball altogether. I'm not getting anything from it socially, and my knee is not getting better.

With a renewed focus, I set about getting myself back into my healthy routine.

Food

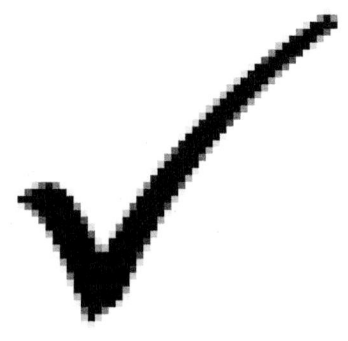

Exercise

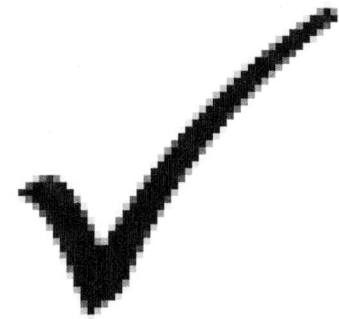

Work/Study

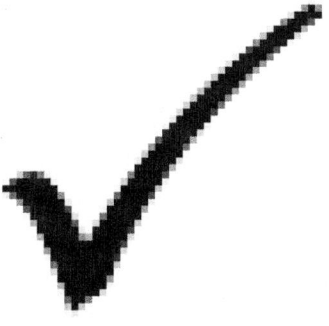

Relationships

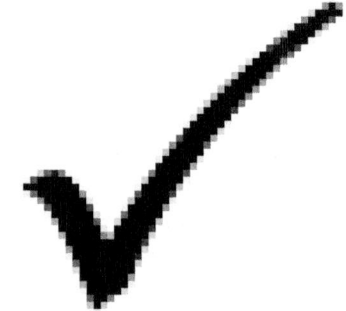

To be in a healthy routine in time for Samuel and my trip away to Wales.

Hoping and praying that this time he will ask me.

Despite being there for a reunion with his undergraduate friends.

We spend two days with his friends.

He then takes me to Snowdonia.

That wasn't what he told me he had planned.

We arrive at a hotel at the base of Cader Idris … which he tells me we are walking up tomorrow.

He knows I love trekking.

That morning he tells me to wait outside whilst he packs his bag.

He takes a hikers rucksack whereas I just take a standard backpack.

Suspicious much.

We stop near the top for lunch.

He is nervous.

He asks if I want my hot chocolate.

Holly: 'No I'm okay.'

We eat our sandwiches.

He gives me my flask of hot water and a spoon with Belgian hot chocolate on it.

Samuel: 'I know you liked that hot chocolate when we were in Bruges.'

Hmmm

I stir it then lift the spoon up.

There's still chocolate on it,

Samuel: 'Lick it.'

Holly: 'No, I don't eat chocolate. I only have hot chocolate.'

Samuel takes the spoon and licks it.

Passes it back to me.

I look at it. Read it in fact.

I look up at Samuel.

He is on one knee with a ring.

Samuel: 'Will you marry me?'

I nod then pull his t-shirt I'm wearing over my head.

I quickly pull it down and cuddle him.

I'm so embarrassed.

I'm his fiancée.

He's asked me to marry him.

He loves me.

Is he mad?

In a state of bliss, we make our descend back to the hotel.

To our room where there are roses waiting for me.

The sheer bliss continues ... for weeks.

It outshines and overshadows everything.

So I don't worry when I continue to eat the flapjack bars I struggled with whilst away.

They are from a health shop after all.

I also don't worry when I find myself in the supermarket after I've been to the gym. Where I buy breakfast bars.

It's only one box ... at a time.

You can stop it. Anytime you like.

But then, just like that I do worry.

I worry because I need to start applying for post-docs. And I am not going to perform well at interviews if I am fat.

I worry because I am about to start refresher driving lessons. Lessons which require full concentration. Concentration I don't have when I am consumed with being fat.

I also worry because the first steps introduction course at the eating disorder service is about to start. Another situation I can't do well in if I have put on weight.

Particularly as it is a re-occurring group session lasting for six whole weeks. And will see people there who are skinner than me.

Not that that will take much.

With no choice I go cold turkey on the bars.

My mood takes a dive.

A further dive when I realise that it's too little too late.

I'm sat in the waiting room with eight other people.

We move to a clinic room.

I rush in so I can pick a seat in the corner.

Not that corners exist in a circle. So I sit furthest away.

It's where I sit for all six sessions.

The six sessions being about everything I know and have heard about before.

But the group is supportive and I'm determined to make the most of this service.

With that in mind, I push for individual therapy at the end of the course, rather than attending the bulimia self-help group that they suggest.

After all, in order to combat it, I need to address the role my BPD plays in maintaining my eating disorder.

CHAPTER 19

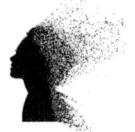

I SUBMIT my PhD within three years of starting it and take a stop-gap job as a locum PWP.

Though okay with my weight therefore okay to face the viva panel, I am the most petrified I have ever been.

Samuel books us a hotel the night before and surprises me by bringing my bedspread and Quentin, my toy duck, to comfort me. But it's not enough. Not enough to stop me dissociating as a way of escape.

Escape from the niggling voice.

The voice that tells me on repeat that I am going to screw it up.

That I am going to fail.

That they are going to laugh me out of the room.

That since I left school, this has all been a big game. A game where I get so far, only for the rug to be pulled from my feet at the last minute.

And it's true.

I can't even answer their first question.

Fuck.

Somehow it's over. I walk out the room and wait whilst they make their decision.

I go back.

Examiners: 'You pass subject to amendments.'

You what?

I walk out dazed.

I stay dazed for the rest of the day.

A week later they call me. They want to change it.

They want to give me extra time to complete the amendments.

Give me twelve months instead of six.

It'll be a re-submission without a viva.

They tell me its' because I'm working full time.

The choice is mine.

Why can't I do anything right the first time?

Not to shoot myself in the foot, I take it.

I take it with a promise to make myself suffer.

To suffer even more after going clubbing with Steven and friends to celebrate our birthday.

Where he tells everybody that I am a Dr.

That he is proud of me.

Shut up. Don't tell me that.

That he, nor the rest of my family thought I would actually be a Dr.

That he thought I would die from the eating disorders.

I'm speechless. Utterly speechless.

CHAPTER 20

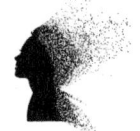

The journey to therapy is often an arduous
one. Flipping between emotions every few
minutes leaves no time for adjustment and
dissection.
Not knowing where I stand with myself
shatters the upcoming performance. Anxiety
mounts as I get nearer to the destination.
One hundred plans flitter through my mind,
but none stay. Requiring a solid plan that
can be well executed leads to memories of my
naivety being constantly reinforced.
By not letting the words or intent touch me,
I am able to continue participation.

━━━

I'm in individual therapy.
    With a counselling psychologist.
    Assumed it would be a clinical psychologist.
    We'll give it a go.

It may work for me.

After all, the other therapists and treatments haven't been able to hit the nail quite on the head.

But I'm worried.

Worried because I haven't made myself sick in months.

Worried because I haven't properly starved myself in years.

Worried because I'm not self-harming or taking overdoses. Not that these things are directly related to an eating disorder.

The only thing I do have is exercising. But I don't do enough for it to qualify as an unhealthy behaviour related to controlling weight.

I tell myself that eating disorders are more than food. They are about feelings.

I tell myself that symptoms change and develop and with that so does diagnosis.

I tell myself that it is not what I look like, it's about how I think.

And finally, I tell myself that it's been thirteen years since my eating disorders kicked off. Seventeen years since I started messing around with food and exercise, and twenty-seven years since I made the link between my body and food.

Surely that's enough to qualify me for treatment.

So, I go into my sessions refusing to be seen as unworthy of treatment.

I go in, firm in my beliefs.

Beliefs about my eating disorder.

Beliefs about my past and current behaviours and thoughts.

Beliefs about their routes.

Beliefs about my childhood.

Beliefs about my family.

Beliefs that I won't budge on. Can't budge on.

Alina says that the current issue is exercising which will be the focus of our work together.

But I'm not doing enough to warrant change.

She tells me that I am over-exercising.

No. Just no.

She suggests keeping a diary.

I'm not keeping another bloody diary. I know what I am doing and as I said it's not enough.

Alina says the diary is not only to note what I am doing, but how it makes me feel.

It doesn't make me feel anything.

I leave the session pissed off. Not that I let it show.

Holly, just do it. See how it goes.

So I do.

Again, I'm compelled to do as I'm told.

I note that at this point I have exercised for eight hundred and twenty five days straight.

I note that on average I go to bed by nine pm.

I note that on average I get up at three am.

I note that every day I do between forty-five minutes and three hours of exercise. Before work. Work being an eight or twelve hour shift five days a week. Work meaning a four hour commute each day. Work also being making amendments to my PhD every evening and at the weekends.

I note that I go to the gym three to four times a week.

I note that I double up on exercising to cover me for days when I am away and may not be able to exercise. Meaning that some days I will do six hours of exercise.

I note that the days I worry I won't be able to exercise, I find myself doing it anyway. Doing sit ups in the bathroom or in the middle of the woods when camping.

I note that I check the gym website to see how long I am there for each session.

I note that I use my Fitbit to track the types of exercises I complete.

I note that every hour my Fitbit goes off to remind me to walk, I will stand on the spot marching.

I note that I have to complete at least ten thousand steps a day. Resulting in me sometimes marching on the spot for half an hour to achieve it, when I can't go out for fear of being seen in public.

Alina asks how it makes me feel.

I don't know what to say.

I don't know if there are any feelings.

It's just something I do.

Something I need to do.

Something I have to do.

I have no choice nor no control in it.

We agree to challenge this.

Me keeping a diary and focusing in on the thoughts and feelings I have.

Alina helping me unpick the reasons behind the compulsion.

Not that I see it as a compulsion or an excessive behaviour.

So I'm surprised when I start to note my thoughts.

Thoughts that I don't actually want to be at the gym.

Thoughts that I don't want to do the home workouts or the HIT exercises.

Thoughts that I actually just want to stay in bed with Samuel.

Yet doing the exercises makes me feel good.

Makes me feel productive.

That I have achieved something.

They set me up for the day.

Exercising also means that I can eat.

Eat without beating myself up.

Eat without the all-consuming thoughts of making myself sick or the desperate desire to cut myself.

It also means that I can be at work and focus on work.

Also focus on finishing my PhD

And most importantly, focus on other people. Particularly Samuel.

Can I really risk my work, PhD and focus on others in the pursuit of stopping exercise?

⸻

It's the first of January 2018.

Alina and I have discussed me asking Samuel for help and support in reducing my exercise.

It means taking a big risk.

A risk in involving somebody else in my eating disorder battle.

A risk of it not working.

A risk of it ruining our relationship.

And a risk of being rejected.

Can't do it today.

Will do it tomorrow.

It's the second of January 2018.

My alarm goes off at two fifty five am.

I'm lying in bed. My mind going round in circles.

I don't want to get up.

I don't want to go to the gym.

I need to go to the gym.

I don't want to go to work.

I need to go to work. I don't get paid otherwise.

If I go to work I need to make a decision about the gym now.

I should ask Samuel.

I can't ask Samuel.

It means waking him up.

What if he gets annoyed at me?

What if he doesn't.

I've already asked him for help. He will be expecting it.

But what if he snaps at me?

He has the rest of the day at home. He can go back to sleep.

Tentatively I reach out to Samuel.

I touch his arm.

I wait for a response.

Nothing.

I touch his arm again. This time a big harder.

I whisper to him.

He responds.

Holly: 'Do I need to go to the gym?'

Samuel: 'No, you don't need to.'

Holly: 'Okay.'

Samuel falls back to sleep straight away.

I lay there.

Thinking.

And thinking.

An hour passes and I'm still in bed. Awake. Wide awake.

Guess I'm not going to the gym.

But I still need to do some exercise.

I get up, do a forty-five minute home workout and a half hour HIT program.

Then I go to work. Not knowing how I feel.

Asking Samuel seems to be a good thing. A really good thing. According to Alina. Not me.

For me it's a sign of being dependent.

A sign of weakness.

And a start of things unravelling.

It's as if asking Samuel that one time has opened a gateway.

A gateway of excuses not to go.

A gateway of where I do not need to take responsibility for the outcome. When the outcome is negative.

A gateway where Samuel is at fault.

And soon enough he is.

Doing as Alina asks, I continue to seek out Samuel's opinion on whether I should go to the gym or not. Mainly on days that I am struggling.

Sometimes he says no. Other times he says it's up to me.

Helpful much.

Soon enough I find myself out of a routine.

And more tired than I have ever been.

With it my mood becomes darker.

I'm pissed off, agitated, frustrated and angry. Really angry.

It gets worse when he switches his mind.

Tells me that I should go to the gym.

Obviously because I am disgusting.

Tells me there is no harm as our wedding is coming up.

He's demanding that I lose weight before the wedding!!

Why? When he has also told me that I need to get my head sorted now we are getting married.

Which is what I am doing. Hence being back in treatment.

I'm starting to go off him, and quite rapidly.

As if he has just realised what he has said, he tells me that he will also come to the gym with me.

That we can go three to four times a week in the morning.

But he will not get up before four am to do so.

So not only is he telling me I need to go to the gym, he is telling me how often and when I can go.

Niggling voice: 'Is this the type of person you want to be with? The type of person you want to marry.'

SHUT UP. SHUT THE FUCK UP.

Samuel is my world. He is my everything. There is no way he would be saying this to hurt me. To try and change me. Mould me to be the person he wants me to be.

So fuck off, RIGHT NOW.

I'm filled with constant anger.

Anger that tells me that I am conforming to him.

Anger that tells me that no matter what I do it is not good enough.

Anger that makes me want to throw it all back in his face.

So I do.

If he doesn't want to get up until four am then fine.

I'll still get up early and simply do more exercises at home.

I'll go to the gym more often and push myself harder to ensure I lose as many calories as I can.

If I end up collapsing or even dying then it's on him. Not me. It's never on me.

I stick to the plan.

So does Samuel. Getting up at four am despite not being a morning person and despite not going to bed till late.

Sometimes letting me drive there in spite of my inexperience and need for his guidance.

I start to think that this new routine could work.

Or not.

I park up at the gym.

He reviews my driving.

Of course he does.

Makes some comments on improvements.

I don't take it well.

He gets stressed.

Slaps his legs and makes frustration noises. Says that he can't do this.

I do not have time for this. We are already behind schedule.

I ask him what's up.

What he wants me to do.

He refuses to get out of the car.

He tells me to leave the car keys with him.

So I get up and leave.

I take my towel and water bottle with me. Tell him I'm leaving my phone and house keys in the boot, as normal.

I go on the cross trainer. Look out the window and watch him in the car.

Watch him drive away.

What the fuck? He is leaving me here, with no way of contacting him or getting back into our flat. What the fuck does he expect me to do?

Fine.

Fuck you.

I don't need you.

Don't even want you.

It's over.

Within ten minutes he is back.

Stays in the car.

Why is he back?

I don't need him.

I'm so glad he is back. I love him.

Why is he just sitting there?

Why doesn't he come in or just go home.

Thirty minutes later he comes into the gym.

Tells me he will leave in twenty minutes as he has to get ready for work.

Scared of causing an argument I tell him that's okay and I'll be out within that time.

Means I can't do everything I need to, but I can do what's remaining at home.

I leave the gym. Get in the car. Ask if he is okay.

Spend the five minute ride home in silence.

Once ready for work, he tells me that he is extremely anxious and that he is sorry for driving off.

I pull faces and try to make him laugh.

We cuddle. Tightly and for a long time.

I really do love him so much.

But I just don't like the way he reacts when he is anxious.

I'm so confused.

Confused enough to bring it up in therapy.

Alina asks what I could have done instead.

Holly: 'Could of taken my phone so I could text him and say that he has my keys. To ask him to drop them off then he can go home instead of waiting for me.'

Alina: 'Apart from the practical things, what else could you of done?'

I sit in silence. Not having a clue.

Alina: 'How about talking to him in that moment about how you were feeling?'

Yea I could. But that would mean spending more time just sitting there, when I was already behind schedule. Plus he was anxious so wouldn't be able to cope with what I said.

She gets me to go over what happened after he drove away from the gym.

And I realise something big. Something transformative.

He came back. Samuel came back for me.

Not only did he come back, he waited for me. Sat in the car. A trapped space. For fifty minutes.

He did that for me.

It hits me like a ton of bricks.

He is breaking the rules I have about people. That they will reject and abandon me.

Samuel's not rejecting me nor abandoning me. In fact, he is putting me above his own needs.

Oh blimey.

With encouragement I reflect this back to Samuel.

He listens and takes it on board. Without judgement.

―――――――

That incident has started a shift.

I find myself opening up more to him.

I notice that it makes me feel better. Makes me feel closer to him.

He also opens up to me.

He tells me he has noticed that therapy is helping me. That he worries that once it is over, I will realise that I don't want to be with him. That I will call off the engagement.

I tell him that the opposite is happening.

That I feel closer to him.

That therapy is helping me realise that communication is at the heart of my issues.

And that an inability to say how I feel and what I think results in self-harming behaviours.

I start to communicate my truth to others.

Particularly about our wedding party after Samuel and I elope.

My anger and upset at Mum and Dad initially refusing to come.

At Julie and Laura 'umming' and 'ahing' at whether to come.

At how I feel Steven is the only family member who has my back. Not a millisecond of doubt, he will be there.

And at my other four siblings who decide point blank not to come to our party.

At the same time my need to exercise reduces.

I stop doubling up on sessions in preparation of being away.

I give myself weekends off from the gym. So I can have a lie in. Stay in bed with Samuel.

Rules and structures in other areas of my life start to lessen.

Sometimes I do not need to wash up as soon as we have eaten.

I don't need to do all the clothes washing or all the household chores.

That I can let Samuel help.

I also stand my ground in being treated badly by others. By those I do not know.

By my new manager who ignores me as soon as I start a new locum position.

At her telling me that she wouldn't of given me the job if she knew that I was taking time off to get married.

So I look for a new locum position.

Hand in my notice a week later.

Ready to start at a different NHS service as soon as I return home as a married woman.

⌷

Family and friends know we are eloping. But not when or where.

Because to marry Samuel, I need to commit to him fully. Give him all my attention. Be present in the moment. And I can't do that, if other people were to know.

So we fly off to Ravello four days before the wedding and stay five days afterwards.

I promise myself that the day we land will mark the end of my nine hundred and ninety seven days of daily exercise.

But no. The urge is too strong.

I'm in the bathroom the morning after we arrive, rushing to do my exercises before Samuel wakes up. Hoping that I can sneak back into bed. Back into his arms.

I succeed for the first day. But not the second.

Second day he tells me to hurry up in the bathroom. Not that he knows what I am doing.

I leave, not having done half of the exercises I need too.

He tells me he is going to jump in the shower.

I finish the exercises in the bedroom.

Just as he walks back in.

Phew.

I hope I can stop when we move to the hotel.

Of course I can't.

The hotel has a gym. An outside gym.

Samuel is fine with me using it.

So I go for a run. Five kilometers.

Haven't done that since I left school.

I also continue my home workouts in the bathroom. Even on the day of our wedding and the morning after.

I do two more five kilometer runs before we leave. In the sweltering heat.

When will this ever stop?

Falling back into my exercise routine as soon as we get home makes me think that it never will.

But it does. The week we are down in Kent for our wedding party.

I do my home workouts in the morning. Only for half an hour maximum.

I don't do any HIT workouts.

I don't feel bad for not making my gym hours up beforehand.

And I don't feel any pressure to make them up afterwards.

This is good right?

But there is one thing that is making me anxious about not exercising.

The actual party.

Having my parents and Julie and Laure there. All of whom didn't want to come in the first place. But had a change of heart. My parents particularly after realising the impact their actions were having on me.

Also having Samuel's family there.

Having my friends there. And Samuels friends. Some of whom I haven't met.

Also not having all my family there.

How can some of my own siblings not come to my wedding party?

I start to worry.

Worry about what people there will think.

Will they like the party?

Will they understand the reason behind us eloping?

Will Samuel's family accept me as a Parry?

Will his friends I haven't met before like me? Think I am good enough for him?

People start to arrive.

I need to welcome them. Of course I want to welcome them, but my G*d am I scared.

A short time later they find their groups and take their picnics and chose where to eat. In the barn, in the hay area, in the orchard or out the back.

I need to mingle. I want to mingle. But where do I go? Who do I see first?

I can't do it. Really can't do it.

I start to pace. Julie notices. Asks if I'm okay. Offers to come up and see people with me.

As we walk past, people stare at me. I smile, hoping that is enough.

Samuel then comes.

We take our picnic and sit with others.

Feeling more confident, I move on. Go to a couple of different groups. On my own.

It's now time for Samuel and I to put our wedding clothes on.

I ask Gemma to help me change.

Laura guards the toilet.

Julie comes out to help.

Steven and Samuel's sister gathers everybody in the barn.

I come out of the toilet in my wedding dress.

I burst into tears.

I can't do this. I can't do this.

People are going to look at me. I just can't.

Julie and Gemma hug me. Laura offers comfort with words.

They then go in.

Samuel and I walk to the front of the barn.

He talks me through it. Holds my hand tightly.

My whole body is shaking. Uncontrollably.

The doors open.

People clap and cheer.

I force myself to look up.

Samuel speaks.

Thanking everyone for coming.

Gives Tori the prize for winning the giant word search.

He introduces our short wedding video.

After it plays, we take to the floor for our first dance.

Samuel talks to me throughout. He tells me it is okay. Tells me that I look beautiful. Tells me to focus on him.

The next song on the jukebox play. Samuel invites people to come up and dance.

They do. Eventually.

I make my excuses and get a drink.

Before I know it, the party is over and it's the next day.

━━━

Fourteen years without any significant physical consequence.

Now I'm about to have a right thyroid lobectomy.

Due to having multinodular goiters.

As a result of years of disordered eating.

Mainly from making myself sick.

I'm petrified.

Petrified because I thought that I was somehow immune to any physical damage from my behaviour.

With my windpipe already suppressed, I'm also petrified that too much damage has been done. That I am not going to get through the operation. Either without further complications or alive.

I'm also petrified that the multi nodular goitres in my left thyroid are also going to grow and will need removing at a later date.

Being all consuming, means I have no room for the additional fear of a complete stop in exercising that will follow the operation.

Never one to run away, I fight the fear as I enter the anaesthesia room.

I wake up in pain.

The surgeons tell me that half my thyroid has been removed.

That it took double the time as it was much bigger than expected.

They also tell me that my vocal cords did not respond to stimulation. That I may have vocal paralysis. Either temporary or permanent.

I stay in hospital for the next two days.

No exercising.

After one thousand and seventy four days, the (dare I say it) compulsion has been broken.

I'm surprisingly fine with it.

I go home to start my two weeks rest.

I struggle to talk, to catch my breath and to swallow.

I spend my days sleeping and hardly eating or drinking.

I constantly think of exercising but have no desire to do it.

Wow.

I attempt to return to work, but leave again when I realise I can't talk for long, struggle to hold my pitch, still have limited movement in my neck and cry from exhaustion.

I go to my follow-up appointments.

My thyroid is cancer free.

Score.

But I have subclinical hypothyroidism and temporary vocal paralysis. Both of which may recover.

I guess I'm lucky.

⊏━━⊐

The need to recover for my new job in a month makes the decision to leave my current position early, an easy one.

Again, I spend my days sleeping.

And I return back to therapy.

I notice a look from Alina in my first session back. But there's' no comment.

Second session back, a comment is made. And the session finishes early.

Again.

Because I'm physically struggling.

Third session, the comment is explored more.

How and why have I fallen so quickly back into restrictive eating.

Holly: 'I'm just struggling after the operation.'

Convinced there's something more there, I'm sent away to really think what this could be.

I talk to Samuel about it.

He also think there's something more to it.

I don't. Really don't.

Until I start writing things down.

Holly to Alina: 'Okay, so I really did think that it was the operation hindering my ability to eat. After all, I didn't chose or plan to stop eating. But I THINK, that I'm now using it as an excuse to continue not eating.'

We start to explore what it could be.

Needing people to see that I am hurting. That I am suffering and am in distress. A way for me to ask for help without having to say the words for fear of rejection.

To control something I have no control over.

To punish myself for causing myself damage. For having screwed my life up. For making people go through this with me. For not being perfect.

Thinking there is something wrong with me. That I am not good enough.

Not worthy enough. Not loveable enough. And needing to change myself as a result.

We try to link it to my past.

Being unable to understand my emotions and feeling that I couldn't talk about them to anyone.

Growing up in a big and chaotic family. Being one of eight children and having two half-brothers and two half-sisters who did not like each other. And to all intent and purposes, still don't.

Mum's attention being split across all the children and my Dad.

Dad and my sister having Asperger's. Witnessing the frustration this caused my Mum, particularly with my Dad.

Being labelled as the child with an attitude problem who is naive, has no common sense and is gullible.

Witnessing Mum and Dad being unhappy in their relationship. Particularly seeing Mum have a go at Dad who just sat there and took it.

Constantly being compared to Steven from play-school until we left school aged eighteen.

Then it hits me.

It's my existence.

My eating disorders are my existence.

My ED keeps me safe when I feel most vulnerable.

My ED allows me to manipulate myself to fit in to what I perceive other people want and need.

My ED stops me from feeling emotions that I am uncomfortable and incapable of dealing with.

My ED gives me a purpose. A reason for living.

But it doesn't does it?

It's actually causes me harm. Enough harm to need an operation.

Oh G*d. The one thing that I thought protected me, is the one thing that can cause me the most harm.

I need to let it go.

But how when the eating disorder is me?

It's not Holly and the eating disorder.

It's Holly the eating disorder.

A small but very important distinction.

I know I need to up my food intake.

I tell Alina and Samuel that I will.

But I've got graduation in a month.

I can't have another bad graduation photo.

Not for a fourth time.

And I can't suddenly start eating when comments have already been made about me not eating lunch by people in my new job.

Eating there will just make me anxious which will make me socially inept.

I can't have that.

No Holly.

People won't care or think twice that you start eating.

Don't let what they may think or may not think impact your mental and physical health.

It's been fourteen years.

It's time to overcome this. Once and for all.

Please.

I start by eating a small portion at dinner.

I then start eating lunch.

A piece of fruit.

A couple pieces of fruit.

A small salad.

I head to Bournemouth for graduation.

With Samuel.

Not Mum and Dad who can't make the commute.

And not with Steven who has caught a bad cold.

I cry the night before the ceremony.

Cry because I feel that my family don't care for me. Don't

love me enough to come down.

I cry even though I now see that this is not true.

I cry because I realise that Samuel is with me and that he will always be with me.

I cry because it is okay to let my emotions out, no matter how irrational or rational they are.

I wake and have breakfast on the day of graduation.

Having not eaten breakfast for months.

Samuel surprises me with a card and gifts.

My family text, wishing me the best.

I change into my outfit. I don't feel fat.

We head to the ceremony where I robe up and have my photo taken.

I feel different.

I take my seat.

Head up on stage when my name is called then return to my seat.

I meet Samuel after.

He has a message from Steven.

The message being that he is proud of me.

Shut up! I hate people telling me that.

I turn my phone on.

I'm inundated with messages from my family in the group chat.

They watched the ceremony online.

Screenshot me up there.

Julie made a meme.

We then meet Grace for drinks and dinner.

I feel different because I am different.

I have achieved my goal of being a Dr in psychology.

I am married to a man who loves me and who I love.

And will love forever.

No doubt about that.

We have our own place.

And we now have a tortoise!

But more than this, I am starting to realise that my family do care for me. They do love me.

They always have done.

It may not of been the way I needed it or wanted it when I was younger, but it was there.

It still is there.

I also have friends. Good friends.

With this knowledge comes feelings of being worthy.

Loveable.

Wanted.

Accepted.

All the things I thought my eating disorders was giving me.

But it wasn't.

It was keeping me from them.

So now it's time.

Time to say goodbye.

Goodbye to therapy.

Goodbye to the eating disorder.

EPILOGUE

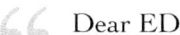 Dear ED,

Writing down what you have taken from me is so hard when you constantly feed me with what good you have done.

Both being aware that your expiration date is fast approaching, a focus on your negatives must prevail.

So here is a list of the pain, the loss, the destruction you have caused, but most of all the reasons for your (soon to be) fall.

You've taken over me so all my senses are consumed by you.

You fill me with crippling self-doubt and self-hatred

You make me question everyone's motives. My trust no longer lies with people, it lies with you.

You've made me an expert in creating extreme anxiety stories based on my deepest vulnerabilities

You've stumped my ability to communicate with others for you are all I think about.

You ensure I doubt my ability in everything I do

You've created fear of certain words that are used as positives and negatives towards me.

You've turned my mood into something that is not representative of who I am.

You have slowly chipped away at me to the point where I truly struggle with everyday tasks.

Worst of all, you've become so entrenched into my psyche that you have become my identity - portraying me as someone I am not and do not want to be.

So, ED what now?

Now it is time that I said goodbye. This time for good. Granted you have been there for me when I had no-one to turn too. But now, I need to venture out into the world on my own. I no longer want to live my life through or for other people. I simply want to live for me. I want to face the world, battle any challenges that may present themselves, and feel all the emotions that there is to feel.

It is time to come out of hiding, to experience both rain and sunshine on my face. It is time that I put full trust, love and care into myself.

It is time to let go of the past and simply live in the moment.

So for now, with a somewhat heavy heart, I say goodbye to you.

(Hopefully, no longer) Yours,

Holly

ABOUT THE AUTHOR

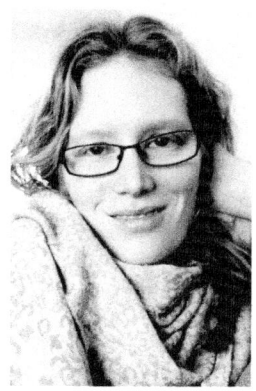

Holly's passion for mental health and helping people has led her to achieve a PhD in psychology and become a psychological wellbeing practitioner.

Currently working as a lecturer in psychology with a specialism in mental health, her research interests include perinatal mental health and the secondary effects of long-term conditions in under-represented groups.

Seeing beauty in vulnerability, Holly strongly believes in using expertise through experience to inspire and empower those she teaches and works with.

With authenticity at its heart, her debut book 'Coming to Terms with Reality' shows that mental illness need not be a barrier to achieving your dreams.

When not working, Holly enjoys spending time with her

growing family, going to the gym, and reading. Sunday mornings she can often be found relaxing at her local coffee shop with friends, family or a good book.

Printed in Great Britain
by Amazon